Patients, Doctors and Healers

Dorthe Brogård Kristensen

Patients, Doctors and Healers

Medical Worlds among the Mapuche
in Southern Chile

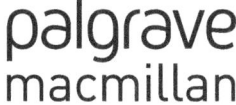

Dorthe Brogård Kristensen
University of Southern Denmark
Odense M, Denmark

ISBN 978-3-319-97030-1   ISBN 978-3-319-97031-8   (eBook)
https://doi.org/10.1007/978-3-319-97031-8

Library of Congress Control Number: 2018959853

This Palgrave Macmillan imprint is published by the registered company Springer Nature
Switzerland AG
The registered company address is: Gewerbestrasse 11, 6330 Cham, Switzerland

ACKNOWLEDGEMENTS

The road to completing this work has been enriching, demanding and often very bumpy. My ambition was to explore the everyday stories and experiences of those people in Chile whose struggle to make sense of their lives had such a profound impact on me. These collective experiences represented a huge accumulation of unarticulated impressions and feelings, apparently stored and ignored until the moment someone chose to address them. In that sense, this task has been very easy, almost like falling down a tube, as someone described the course of my fieldwork. However, fieldwork among medical doctors, Mapuche healers and patients was also quite challenging in that I had to find a way to navigate these unexplored experiences and, not least, to communicate them through academic writing. The field itself also presented many barriers, both due to state bureaucracy, which made access to the public health setting very restricted, and because in what is referred to as the Mapuche world, advocated by political organizations, I was faced by certain barriers. On the one hand, as a European anthropologist I could be a resource in the struggle to claim their rights, but on the other, I was also subjected to the criticism of "intruding" into their authentic culture. In order to support the struggle of those who claim to be "oppressed objects", I often felt that I lost my own sense of agency and the possibility to articulate myself freely. I returned from the fieldwork with the feeling of having, in some way, fragmented into bits and pieces that took several years to glue back into an integrated unit. Therefore, the Mapuche culture per se (if such an entity exists) did not become the focus of this study; rather, the work documents the everyday lives of those people who simply live them, without claiming a political voice for their experiences. I am relieved at having come this far and grateful for all the help and encouragement I received on my way.

This work would not have been possible without the help of many people, foremost being the medical practitioners therein, Dr Luis Silva, Maria Angelica Parra, Sebastián Allilef and José Caripan, without whose openness and generous sharing of knowledge I could not have embarked on this study. I also thank the Mapuche pharmacy and the hospital of Temuco for permitting me to observe medical consultations. Special thanks go to all the patients in this study, who so generously opened their homes and hearts to the anthropologist. Also, thanks to José Aylwin, the lawyer who gave me an insight into the world of indigenous rights, first at the Universidad de la Frontera, and afterwards at the non-government organization Observatorio de los Derechos de los Pueblos Indigenas.

This study was made possible with funding from the Humanistic Research Council. Here I also want to mention those who originally inspired me to take up this work. At the Department of Anthropology at the University of Copenhagen, Cecilie Rubow and my supervisor for my master's thesis, Hanne Veber, both encouraged me to embark on this project. Another source of inspiration came from the insights provided by Bruce Kapferer, Murray Last and Roland Littlewood during my stay between 1997 and 1998 at University College, London.

My PhD supervisors, Karsten Pærregård and Helle Johannessen, always provided me with inspiration and the encouragement to get the dissertation into shape. I also thank the PhD group in the Department, not least Jens Kofoed, Kristina Wimberly, Mette Ringsted and Charlotte Jacobsen, for their continuous support and feedback on my writing. I owe a great debt to Mark Vacher and Kåre Jansbøl for inspiration, support and for reading and commenting on drafts, and I would especially like to thank my friends for their continuous encouragement and support in the writing up of this work: among these are Mette Kyung Reacroft, Ann-Dorte Hass Jensen, Desirée Aurora Nielsen, Nanna Ahlmark, Helle Jensen, Lene Okholm, Vibeke Emborg and Martin Lindhardt in Denmark and, to mention only a few, Hellen Pacheco, Anita Millarey, Eliseo Huencho, Mabel García, Willi Collipal, Kamilla Karen Collipal and Maria Velasquez in Chile.

I owe Ana Mariella Bacigalupo a debt of gratitude for the scholarly inspiration gained through reading her work, and for contacting me and encouraging me to turn my dissertation into a book, and Alexis Nelson for providing me with the contact at Palgrave. I also thank Jennifer Guzman, encountered at an AAA conference, for giving me guidance. In revising my original work and turning it into a book, the advice of Benedikte Møller Kristensen, Charlotte Bredahl Jacobsen, Vibeke Nielsen and the comments from Pablo Marimán have been of huge value. Special warm thanks also go to Marie-Louise Karttunen for her careful reading of the whole manuscript.

Thanks are owed to my mother Lizzi, to Christian, and especially to my son Lican for his patience in adapting to two realities in the first years of his life: one in a flat in the centre of Copenhagen with his mother, another in a house below the scenic Villarica volcano on an indigenous reservation living among shamans, Mapuche and his father's relatives. Thank you for being wise and lively company through all this journey.

CONTENTS

LIST OF FIGURES

CHAPTER 1

Illness Stories, Medical Choices and Socio-Political Process

This book explores notions of culture, identity and power in the bodily experiences and medical choices of patients in Southern Chile. The ethnographic material consists of case stories of patients, both Mapuche and mestizo, who combine biomedical treatment with the traditional medicine of the Mapuche. During recent decades the practice of Mapuche healers—shamans and herbalists—has been revitalized and become a very popular medical choice among Mapuche and mestizo, especially near urban centres (Bacigalupo 2001). With a population of about 1.7 million or about 10% of the total population, the Mapuche constitute the largest ethnic minority in modern Chile.[1] Most Chileans, however, refer to themselves as mestizo, which means that they have mixed indigenous and European roots.

The main question explored is why actors perceive a certain medicine as effective, a question born out of my observation that health problems—as well as the knowledge and experience of illness and the use of medicines—were often-discussed topics among members of the family, neighbours and colleagues. Such conversations frequently touched upon illnesses that involved symptoms with no apparent organic pathology; in particular, people shared stories of "strange" afflictions with quite similar symptoms. Typically these included psychological symptoms like anxiety, lack of energy, loss of memory and a constant desire to cry, combined with diffuse physical symptoms such as dizziness, nausea, swellings or intense pain;

---

[1] http://www.censo2017.cl/wp-content/uploads/2018/05/presentacion_de_la_segunda_entrega_de_resultados_censo2017.pdf.

© The Author(s) 2019
D. B. Kristensen, *Patients, Doctors and Healers*,
https://doi.org/10.1007/978-3-319-97031-8_1

1

most often manifested in the head or stomach, they also had a tendency to move location within the body. Some cases discussed, however, also involved serious, and often terminal, diseases which had a biomedical diagnosis; the most common was cancer.

In these stories people also reported strange incidents in their houses, mentioning things that had started to disappear, move around or simply crack. Some heard footsteps and felt watched by a presence. Others commented that they were not feeling like themselves, that they often lost control of their body, typically their tongue or legs, and some even felt that an alien presence had physically invaded them (often depicted as an insect or a lizard, which then fed off the body). These stories were accompanied by complaints that recent social changes and modernity in general had not brought much that was good, while many people expressed a general feeling of being stuck in a rut without many opportunities to change the current social and economic situation. Others said they felt "crushed" and that they did not feel "alive". In addition, people complained of the cost of biomedical treatment and the long wait to be examined, as well as the frequent failure of biomedical doctors to detect a disease. A fundamental part of these stories was the evaluation they contained of the medical diagnosis and treatment that the patients had received from their biomedical doctors, as well as Mapuche healers.

The underlying assumption of this work, stemming from observations expressed in these conversations, is that these medical dialogues encapsulate issues that do not relate only to health problems; notions of power and identity in relation to social and political processes also seem to be implied. In their work on multiple personality disorder, Ian Hacking and Paul Antze argue that categories have the capacity to "make up" people (Hacking 1995, 1996; Antze 1996). In a social context categories take on a life of their own; they become entities which people come to inhabit, and through which they invoke meaning in their lives (Antze 1996: 3). Antze further poses the following question: What happens to people who come to live inside a discourse, who use it to make sense of their life? One way of answering this question, he suggests, is by analysing the stories that people tell about themselves, arguing that even trivial anecdotes can be considered highly interesting when told in the course of social interaction. He consequently proposes that stories "might be the chief means by which grand cultural discourses like Christianity or psychoanalysis find their way into something resembling self-knowledge" (Antze 1996: 6); in other words, stories reflect how people experience, articulate and negotiate the self and personhood in relation to the languages available in a given context.

The bodily afflictions encompassed in this work, which are shared in medical dialogues and diagnosed by patients and practitioners within alternative or indigenous medical traditions, have been referred to as "folk illnesses", idioms of distress (Nichter 1981; Kaiser et al. 2015) or "culture-bound syndromes" (Simons and Hughes 1985) in the anthropological and biomedical literature (Panter-Brick and Eggerman 2017). Locally they are referred to as Mapuche illnesses or spiritual illnesses, as alternative and Mapuche practitioners often explain illnesses through the Mapuche worldview. Indigenous disease categories are part of a general repertoire of folk knowledge. Here the distinction between, on the one hand, natural illness, such as colds, wounds, infections and flu, and, on the other, spiritual (or supernatural) illness reflects popular talk on health matters. To the latter category of spiritual illness belong those types of afflictions in which an external agent—a spirit, ancestor or witch—is believed to have affected both the body of the patient and his or her surroundings, causing physical, psychological and social imbalances.

I was puzzled by the fact that many urban modern citizens—mestizo and Mapuche—diagnosed and treated themselves with Mapuche medicine for "strange" afflictions, the so-called Mapuche illnesses or spiritual illnesses. Did they have a biomedical condition which the doctors had not discovered? Or was something else going on? And what happened in those cases where patients actually did have a biomedically diagnosed disease, but still insisted they had a spiritual or a Mapuche illness? Consequently, the aim of this book is to explore stories of folk or Mapuche illness by following the patients' articulation and management of afflictions in a context in which both the diagnosis and treatment take place within a pluralistic medical system: in other words, where the patient attends a variety of practitioners such as doctors, psychiatrists and Mapuche healers. The patient might accept a biomedical diagnosis of cancer while at the same time consulting a shaman in search of both the cause of, and the cure for, the illness, indicating that the patient holds a pluralistic and complex view of his or her identity, culture and body. In this way medical choices and dialogue can serve as a lens through which complex identities and social and political processes can be analysed.

WHO CURED WANGLEN?

The case of Wanglen,[2] a young Mapuche girl, serves to raise some of the issues explored in this book, meanwhile illustrating my navigation in the field between medical practitioners, patients and their therapy management groups. Wanglen's case is interesting, both because her illness was familiar to many people in the area and therefore often discussed and commented upon by patients I met during my fieldwork, and also because it challenges a common assumption within anthropology that folk illness is primarily connected to psychological and social distress (Nichter 1981; Rubel et al. 1984). Wanglen lived with her parents in a rural area about one hour away from Temuco. Her parents were Mapuche and quite successful, working as consultants for a governmental programme for indigenous peoples. Wanglen was, at the time of my fieldwork in 2004, a 6-year-old girl who had suddenly collapsed and entered a state of coma, although at first nobody knew the cause of her strange condition. I first heard of the case from a herbalist, Maria, who worked at the medical centre of a Mapuche pharmacy in Temuco. She told me that Wanglen's parents had arrived at her consultation in the medical centre the day after the girl had become comatose, when Wanglen was hospitalized in the intensive care unit (ICU) for children in the hospital in Temuco.

Maria had visited the girl in the hospital and, by touching her pulse, had diagnosed her as suffering from *trafentun*—also referred to as susto—which occurs when the soul or vital force has been captured by spirits, or when a part of the soul has been lost due to a startling or frightening event. Maria was sure that the soul of the girl could be recovered with Mapuche medicine and that she could, thereby, be healed, but that as a herbalist (*lawentuchefe*) she herself did not have sufficient spiritual power to undertake the cure, since her expertise was in medicinal plants, not in the rituals that are necessary to regain parts of the soul that had been lost. She gave Wanglen an antidote (*contra*) and a cleansing medicine (*sahumerio*), but recommended that Wanglen's parents consult a powerful shaman by the name of Sebastian, who also worked in the medical centre of the Mapuche pharmacy. The parents never arrived at Sebastian's consultation, however, and nor did they finish the herbalist's treatment; therefore Maria asked me to help find out what had happened to the girl.

---

[2] The names of the medical practitioners and the girl Wanglen have not been altered, but names given for other patients are pseudonyms.

Four months later, when I was conducting participant observation in the local hospital, I had the opportunity to visit the ICU. I was surprised to find that Wanglen was still there, but no longer in a state of coma; rather, I found a very pretty, lively, smiling girl in a wheelchair. Her parents approached me somewhat suspiciously, but when I told them that I knew Maria they willingly told me their daughter's illness story. Wanglen had been playing ball and suddenly collapsed on her way to the toilet and subsequently went into a state of coma, which required a respirator and intravenous feeding for four months. After her hospitalization the girl was subjected to a range of examinations, including blood, urine and stool tests and checks on her veins and for possible ulcers; samples were also sent to the USA for testing. The biomedical doctors who treated Wanglen eventually diagnosed her as suffering from Guillain-Barré syndrome, explained as a virus that, without warning, attacks and paralyses muscles and nerves to such a degree that the patient stops breathing.

Wanglen's parents accepted the medical diagnosis, but they did not consider it sufficient or complete in that no medicine or treatment was provided, apart from the technologies for prolonging the girl's life. They wanted to take her to a specialist in the USA, but gave up the idea due to lack of funds. After the consultation with Maria they decided to consult the shaman José Caripan, who had been recommended by people they knew at home. Apart from susto, José also diagnosed Wanglen as suffering from *mal* (*kalkutun*), an affliction produced by a sorcerer through the poisoning of food, beverages or objects.

Both Maria and José Caripan said, independently, that the girl had encountered negative energy on that day when she was playing outside her home, and this had caused her present situation. Both practitioners also said that the girl would recover, and their prophecy turned out to be correct. In fact, according to her parents, Wanglen returned to consciousness on the same day they consulted José Caripan, which, they felt, was sure proof of the effectiveness of Mapuche medicine. At the hospital the staff had been very attentive to the girl, and they had succeeded in keeping her alive with their technological devices: the respirator and feeding tubes. In the opinion of Wanglen's parents, however, the biomedical doctors were not responsible for her cure.

I also interviewed the doctor who treated Wanglen. She was a tall, blonde woman (indicating European descent) who did not share the parents' opinion, nor did she seem at all moved by the miracle of Wanglen's recovery. Saying that she preferred to speak with me privately, she invited me into her office and closed the door, whereupon she pronounced, "I'd rather speak frankly from the start; I am anti-Mapuche." She observed with some irritation that the government had given land to the Mapuche near her residence, "And the only thing that they did with the land was to cut down all the trees; apart from this they did nothing. In my view, the Mapuche culture represents nothing of value." I did not go into the details of this statement, merely asking her opinion of Wanglen's recovery. She began by complaining that it had been extremely difficult to get the parents' cooperation in their daughter's treatment. The most serious disagreement, however, had arisen over the question of which medicine cured Wanglen, with the doctor commenting bitterly, "I bet Wanglen's mother goes around saying that Mapuche medicine cured her daughter, but we were the only ones who ever did anything for that child. Without us she would never have been cured." I told her that Wanglen's mother had expressed gratitude for the hospital's openness to, and acceptance of, their giving their daughter Mapuche medicine. "Yes," she said, "we just let them give it to her; it could not do much harm. I believe they are communists. How to put up with people like that?"

Complex Illnesses, Complementary Cures

Wanglen's case and diagnostic process highlight a number of relevant themes and problems that are central to this book, first and foremost the complex reality of medical pluralism, of which both patients and practitioners form part. Wanglen's parents apparently accepted the diagnosis of all the practitioners they consulted, so this case could be regarded as an example of complementary medicine and the parallel diagnosis and treatment that were quite prevalent in the context of Southern Chile. But why did they insist on the effectiveness of Mapuche medicine at the expense of biomedicine? This leads back to the important question of why actors perceive a certain medicine to be effective.

Chilean doctors know that many patients explain their afflictions on the basis of what the medical profession refers to as the "animistic beliefs of the patients", the term for the indigenous belief that external agents and moral transgressions cause bodily conditions. Most doctors, however, regard these beliefs as folk superstition dating back to the era before modernization and industrialization turned Chile into a modern nation-state. "There is nothing wrong with them, they just feel awful," remarked a Chilean doctor of the health problems that afflict what he estimates as around 70% of his patients.

This was his way of expressing his annoyance with, and scepticism of, the number of patients who complained of aches and pains, swellings, anxiety, lack of energy and sadness, among other symptoms, which do not really fall within the ambit of a general practitioner, as no organic pathology can be detected. Doctors are also aware that most patients still use alternative and indigenous medicine and that many believe they have a spiritual or Mapuche illness. When a "real" organic disease is apparent, some doctors simply prohibit the combination of different types of medicine, while others allow the patients to combine biomedicine with "natural" or Mapuche medicine, not because they believe it might be effective, but because they feel that it "probably won't do much harm". This applies to symptoms that the biomedical literature defines as psychosomatic or "medically unexplained symptoms"[3] (Kirmayer 2004), or, as one doctor put it, "imagined illnesses". If these illness problems are considered at all a case for a biomedical practitioner, then psychiatrists and psychologists are expected to deal with them. Most biomedical doctors diagnose these afflictions as depressions, states of anxiety or simply nerves (*sistema nerviosa*). Another smaller group of patients is treated for cancer or irritable bowel syndrome, the latter suffering which many doctors suspect to be psychosomatic.

While patients diagnosed with organic diseases, such as cancer patients, receive proper treatment, the majority without a "real" diagnosis are left untreated by the health system, as departments like psychiatry, psychology and neurology have very limited resources at their disposal. The doctor who claimed that 70% of his patients had nothing wrong with them—in common with the other doctors who participated in this study—was also resigned to the fact that many, if not all, of these patients combined biomedical treatment with the use of other medicine due to their "animistic" beliefs. Doctors were also resigned to the circumstance that other types of medicine provided an explanation for both the physical and psychological symptoms of the patients. In any case, a viewpoint accepted by all is that the public health system does not have sufficient resources to cover the demand.

Turning to the world of the patients, a completely different scenario unfolds. While doctors might find that "nothing is wrong" or alternatively offer a biomedical diagnosis of psychiatric disorder, many patients do not

---

[3] According to Lawrence Kirmayer, the term "medically unexplained symptoms" names a social and clinical predicament, not a specific disorder. He furthers argues that many cultural traditions provide socio-somatic theories, which link social conditions with physical symptoms and illnesses (Kirmayer 2004: 663).

accept either type of explanation for their affliction for very long. In the medical context of Chile, numerous healing practices exist which offer disease categories, explanations of symptoms and, most importantly, possible cures. Thus, the context is characterized by both biomedicine and multiple parallel healing practices, among which is the so-called Mapuche medicine practised by shamans (machis) and herbalists (*meicas* and *lawen-tuchefe*). In addition, various imported healing practices exist such as Bach medicine, acupuncture and spiritualist healing. In this work I focus on the two most used in Southern Chile: biomedicine and Mapuche medicine.

In their medical work, Mapuche practitioners normally diagnose on the basis of examining a patient's urine (*willintun*) or touching his or her pulse; other ways of diagnosing are by touching the patient's clothes (*pewuntun*) or through dreams (*pewma*). Treatment consists of a combination of rituals and herbal remedies. It is, however, mostly the machis who use rituals in their medical treatment, which they combine with a trance state that is used both for diagnosis and for curing. Many Mapuche practitioners consider themselves Christians—Catholic or evangelical—and integrate Christian symbols and saints into their medical work.

MAPUCHE ILLNESS AS A SOCIAL, CULTURAL AND POLITICAL ARENA

Wanglen's parents' combination of different strategies and medical options both taps into a set of worldviews that conflict with Western medicine, as well as highlighting a class and ethnic struggle. This was especially apparent in their conflict with the doctor over Wanglen's recovery: in the end, who cured Wanglen? There is no simple answer to this question and no way to identify what really helped her to recover; as with the aetiology of the mysterious affliction, these are issues that could never be resolved. Relevant here is the question of why certain types of cultural, socio-economic and political realities produce certain types and manifestations of illness.

At first sight, the case of Wanglen's susto could be regarded as an example of those cases which, in the anthropology and cultural psychiatry literature, have been referred to as culture-bound syndromes, also to be found in an appendix to the Diagnostic and Statistical Manual of Mental Disorders (DSM IV). Susto has been widely interpreted as social role stress (Rubel et al. 1984). However, Wanglen's case challenges some of the common assumptions, both in medical practice and the literature, about culture-bound syndromes because, firstly, she actually had an organic and biomedical diagnosis. Her susto could hardly be described as psychological or simply imagined. Another interesting question in this connection, also raised by Libbet Crandon-Malamud (1983), is why a child would be diagnosed as suffering from Mapuche illness or a culture-bound syndrome. The diseases of children challenge the assumption of both biomedical doctors and the literature that Mapuche illnesses or folk illnesses are mainly "matters of the mind" and a way for those on the margins of society to articulate social distress. It seems a bit far-fetched to conclude that a 6-year-old child would express social role stress in this manner. Nonetheless, this interpretation of culture-bound syndromes, among which susto figures, has been widely accepted within the literature and medical practice in Chile. A central argument here, however, is that the appearance of folk illness or culture-bound syndromes is not only a matter of "culture", but is also embedded in struggles of an ideological, cultural and political character. In this way the use of indigenous disease categories and medical practice reflects, as Wanglen's case shows us, struggles of a social and political character, within a system characterized by social inequalities and uneven resources. It is also a struggle of an ideological and cultural kind, relating to the difficulties of defining and dealing with the forces that guide and influence human beings.

FIELD SETTING AND FIELDWORK

The empirical focus of this work is Southern Chile, with a starting point in the town of Temuco, which means "the water of Temu" in the Mapuche language (called *mapudungun*); it is also the name of a medicinal plant used by the Mapuche. The town is regarded as the heart of what was formerly known as the Mapuche nation and is characterized by the presence of the Auracanians—or the Mapuche, as they are referred to today. According to official national history, the Mapuche fought tirelessly and fearlessly against the Incas and the Spanish for 300 years, their indigenous lands only becoming part of Chile after 1884. The founding of Temuco, part of a military strategy to colonize the south, took place in 1881 after a bloody battle, whereupon the indigenous population was assigned territories (*communicades*). The colonization of Temuco is one chapter of a violent and traumatic history; the military regime of Augusto Pinochet from 1973 to 1989, which sought to "erase the Marxist cancer", comprises another. The latter was a serious blow against any political action or movement that could be regarded as Marxist, as well as the political rights of the Mapuche, as their original territories were privatized and in many cases transferred to multinational timber companies with the goal of spurring economic growth.

Today Temuco is an important administrative, industrial and tourist centre, has about 400,000 inhabitants and is considered one of the fastest-growing cities in Latin America. It also has the greatest concentration of Mapuche (23%) in Chile, as well as the highest percentage of people living below the poverty line, which during the time of fieldwork in some areas was more than 59%.[4] Temuco is the centre of the Mapuche political movement, which, since the introduction of democracy in 1989, has struggled for the political recognition of the Mapuche as a people as well as for the recovery of indigenous territories. Since the implementation of an Indigenous Law (Ley Indigena 19.253) in 1993, some parts of the original indigenous territories have been returned and transferred to indigenous owners.

The fieldwork took place over 12 months during 2004–2005 in Southern Chile, in a context of medical pluralism. The aim of my fieldwork was to engage with medical practitioners and their patients, within the fields of both biomedicine—in this case the public health system—and Mapuche medicine. Methodologically, I take my cue from the Manchester School. With Max Gluckman as its prime inspiration, the Manchester School developed the ethnographic extended-case method, also known as situational analysis, with the ambition of arriving at the general through a dynamic particularity of the specific or the case (Gluckman 1958, 2006; van Velsen 1967; Kapferer 1987, 2006; Turner 1957, 1967). The focus of the case study is on the complex interplay between social relationships and the choices of individuals, and between institutions and customs (Kempny 2006). The method of the Manchester School was very appropriate to my research design, firstly due to the apparent practicality of the method in working with a defined analytical unit, and secondly because I shared the theoretical ambition of linking a specific observed case with social and political processes in order to arrive at general hypotheses or theories. I was also interested in studying the networks of actors—from political institutions, through health sectors, to indigenous communities—meaning that the study required an ethnography of diverse contexts.

I made use of both the event and the patients as case material. The event is defined as medical consultations in the context of medical pluralism; that is, the consultations of biomedical doctors and Mapuche practitioners,

[4] This figure is from the city of Puerto Savedraa (Diario Austral 5 July 2001).

which became my entrance to the field of medical pluralism. The focus of fieldwork was on the social relations involved in the patient's articulation and management of illness: with medical practitioners, family, neighbours, friends and colleagues, or what John Janzen has called the "therapy management group" (1978). I followed patients whom I had first met in medical consultations in their interactions with their social network and during the treatment process. After consultations I visited the patients and their families in their private homes.

IN THE FIELD

Being an anthropologist working with Mapuche is not an easy task and I was often warned that my topic might create mistrust and hostility. I also heard it said that anthropologists are like vampires who suck the knowledge from the Mapuche in order to publish books and get rich (see also Bacigalupo 2007: 30). From the outset of my fieldwork I was really surprised and happy to be allowed to work with the El Centro Medico—the medical centre—of the recently opened Mapuche pharmacy in the centre of Temuco,[5] chosen for its popularity. Here I conducted participant observation from August to October 2004 with two Mapuche practitioners (Maria and Sebastian). In terms of observing consultations and meeting patients, this choice was very successful; my notebook was soon filled with names and phone numbers of patients all wanting to share their illness story and accounts of their "favourite" Mapuche medical practitioners. The interest and openness were overwhelming. However, while both the practitioners and patients there were interested in participating, after two months of fieldwork I was prohibited by the director of the medical centre from continuing my work there, as it had been decided that the work of an anthropologist "does no good to Mapuche medicine".[6] This came as a surprise to me, but was not a real challenge to my research plan, as I had scheduled work with several Mapuche healing practitioners. I then turned to the public health setting.

[5] Since my fieldwork, the Mapuche pharmacy has developed into a chain with a nationwide presence.

[6] The director explained that a Chilean anthropologist had recorded the work of machis (including Sebastian) and afterwards published extracts of conversations and prayers without having asked for permission. The board of directors considered suing her for cultural theft and violation of intellectual property rights. I also heard the story from the anthropologist in question, who insisted that all had consented, but had changed their minds after the book was published.

In this setting, however, patients were rarely interested in talking to me, although some of them spent most of the day awaiting their turn. Even when I actively addressed them, they barely responded and looked very suspicious. I contacted an intercultural organization (*amuldungun*) operating as a linguistic service for patients from a Mapuche background in the hope that its staff could help me in exploring how patients move between Mapuche medicine and biomedicine. In a meeting arranged by the leader at which staff and I were present, staff members announced that they were not interested in working with me, as they had only "negative" experiences with anthropologists, who just "left" with information without giving anything in return. Furthermore, they refused to expose the patients as mere "objects of study". My reiterating that the patients might benefit from a study focusing on their perception of health and illness did not help much.

Illustrating the problems of conducting research in the field of biomedicine in Chile were my attempts to interview the biomedical doctor of one the cases from the field who claimed to have been successfully treated by a Mapuche practitioner. When I approached the doctor, he said that I could return the following week at 8 o'clock. I came early on the agreed day, only to wait an hour and a half for his arrival, during which time I overheard the patient next to me telling her neighbour that he had unsuccessfully treated her for an inflammation of the kidneys; afterwards she had been cured of the affliction by a herbalist. When the doctor arrived and I approached him, he shouted, "I don't have any time." I asked him if he could spare ten minutes some other time. "No," he replied and literally slammed the door. Giving up the plan to interview him, I tried to converse with the patient next to me, asking if she was satisfied with the doctor. "No," she replied, "but I cannot get another doctor, so there is nothing to do but continue with him." When I asked if she had seen any other type of practitioner, she replied "No" and turned her face away. This reluctance to discuss their illnesses while in an official health institution was quite common among patients, unless I knew them beforehand or was recommended by a close relative or acquaintance.

My only "successful" contact in the official health setting was with Dr Silva, who was very interested in the study of patients' "construction of illness", as he phrased it, meaning we had a mutual interest in collaboration. He allowed me to sit in during his consultations and to visit the psychiatric ward. Overall, I spent two months at the Temuco hospital. After much effort and due to Dr Silva's openness, I managed to conduct short individual interviews with Dr Silva and hospital staff, including the administrative head of the hospital, psychologists, social workers, nurses, three doctors, the intercultural service and administrative employees. Conversely, when studying Mapuche practitioners, the whole world opened up to me, and I was met with intense eagerness among both patients and practitioners to share their illness stories. Paradoxically, I even met some of the same patients whom I had met in the official health system, although here, in contrast, they were more than willing to talk to the anthropologist. Indeed, I often felt that the field controlled me rather than the opposite, as I was constantly drawn into the sphere of shamanistic practice, while the role of biomedicine was almost non-existent in the illness narratives I collected. It was almost as though people had been waiting years to offer the anthropologist their special account of the miracles of the Mapuche practitioner. Thus, what seemed to connect me to the informant was a mutual interest in documenting the value of Mapuche medicine.

From my observation of "the event", I chose 30 patients whom I followed during my fieldwork, both in their consultation with other medical practitioners, and in their articulation and negotiation of illness with their "therapy management group"; this enabled me to study the role that social relations played in the interpretation and management of illness (Janzen 1978). The aim was to analyse a type of "system", extrapolating from connections between ethnographic portraits of subjects, and the posited relationship of these portraits, to the fate of subjects in other locations (Marcus 1995: 106). Furthermore—following the ideas of the Manchester School—my ambition was to identity relevant issues in the context, thereby connecting the case to more general themes related to social and political processes in Chile. This corresponds with the method applied in a multisited ethnography, which Marcus refers to as "follow the people", where the procedure is to accompany a particular group of subjects, in this case patients of specific medical practitioners. When interviewing the patients, I focused on the notions of body, illness and cultural identity in relation to diagnosis and treatment by their medical practitioners. Here a huge gap soon became evident between the medical perception of doctors and that of their patients. While they shared the same empirical setting, they rarely shared an understanding of illness and treatment.

MEDICAL WORLDS

It is the relation between different perceptions, understandings and misunderstandings of actors in medical systems which is the focus of this present work. I also focus on the socio-political changes in the biomedical health system, which consists of a relatively rundown and ineffective public system mainly in the service of the poor and the elderly, and a parallel, private health system. Unless medical practice is strictly based on Western medicine, it is not officially recognized. One shared characteristic of the patients suffering from folk illnesses lies in their self-description—or that of their therapy management group—as marginal in terms of the Chilean nation-state. In addition, they often articulate the point of view that traditional Mapuche practitioners, in contrast to biomedical doctors, take their problems seriously and also help them deal with their general situation, hence my suggestion that the choice of medicine reflects both an articulation and a negotiation of social values, identity and power relations. When Wanglen's parents expressed their conviction that José Caripan had cured their daughter, they also articulated an experience of a shared social position with the shaman rather than the doctor.

As already noted, one of the principal purposes of the research which resulted in this book was to explore the social and political processes attendant on illness experiences and medical choices; specifically, to locate the articulation of folk illnesses or Mapuche illnesses in their social and political context. The task has not been, therefore, to describe and analyse medicine or healing practice as systems, but, rather, to understand how people combine different types, given that these practices serve as an empirical prism through which to study how people embody and articulate complex notions of identity, culture and power. Medicines are not only material substances which can serve to relieve physical and psychological suffering, they are also powerful social symbols and historical products embedded in the larger socio-economic, political and historical context framing the power struggles on a broader national (and global) scene. When patients follow a particular medical regimen, they are positioning themselves within webs of meanings as well as structures of power.

THEMES OF CULTURAL REPRESSION: THE OLVIDOS OF CHILE

The main argument of this book is that medical practices serve to uncover hitherto unacknowledged realities—what I call olvidos. According to sociologist Tomas Moulian, the concept of olvido refers to the forgetting of an aspect of the past in societies that have suffered extreme, often violent, experiences, but that lack the social framework to express them. I suggest, therefore, that illness experiences serve to uncover realities that are not part of any official political framework. Borrowing from Freud, I call these "uncanny"[7] experiences; that is, an experience that "ought to have remained hidden but has come to light" (1955: 240). Freud argues that traumatic memories of the past can return in peculiar and "uncanny" ways, what the historian Steve Stern calls the "unexplored hearts and minds" aspect of experience (Stern 2006: xx).

Inspired by the work of Bruce Kapferer (2003), I further suggest that medical choices may allude to a perceived fault in the state, thereby constituting "an implicit critique of the state" and consequently "an action corrective of the state" (Kapferer 2003: 124) by highlighting problematic consequences of social and political processes in Chile. While the more political aspects of Chilean and Mapuche history have been thoroughly discussed in the literature, mundane, everyday life has not been addressed apart from a few exceptions (see, for example, Han 2012). An interesting question here concerns how Chileans—indigenous and non-indigenous—relate to these experiences from their collective past. The memory issue is linked to the question of identity, their collective identity as Chileans, their perceptions of who they are. In this connection the current national ideology of the Chilean state does not allow a framework for the articulating of certain experiences. Consequently, I suggest—as also argued by Chilean authors Montecino (1996) and Moulian (1997)—that the Chilean history of identity is based on a collective repression, and to large degree a collective oblivion—or olvido—of its origins.[8]

---

[7] According to Freud, traumatic memories of the past can also return in peculiar and "uncanny" ways. As he writes, "the uncanny is in reality nothing new or alien, but something which is familiar and old-established in the mind and which has become alienated from it only through the process of repression" (Freud 1955: 240). One example is the superstition of the evil eye, the dread that whoever possesses something that is valuable and fragile is susceptible to the envy of others. Another example is the fear that even an intention can do harm, where certain signs are seen as proof that an intention has the potency to damage. The analysis of "the uncanny" is, in the Freudian universe, connected to an animistic concept of the world which involves, among other things, a view of it as inhabited by the spirits of human beings, by the belief in the omnipotence of thoughts and the attribution of "magical power" to outside persons and things, the so-called *mana*.

[8] This ambivalence is symbolized by the hero of the Chilean nation-state, the liberator Bernardo O'Higgins. According to the historical sources, O'Higgins was the son of a Peruvian governor and a woman of unknown origin, although apparently indigenous. He is typical of the ambivalence of Chilean identity history: his origins are problematic as a result of being a racial mixture and an orphan, yet this did not prevent his becoming a national hero (Montecino 1996: 143).

The first olvido, the whitening, was a result of the process of colonization and the question of cultural and national identity, several issues relating to which have already emerged from Wanglen's story. Mestizo children
were the product of relationships between indigenous women and
Europeans, commonly growing up without a father; they were therefore
referred to as *huachos*, that is, orphans or illegitimate children (Montecino
1996: 20). In official frameworks and discourses for the Chilean nation,
these meanings of mestizaje are not articulated. Nevertheless, the political
project of the elite has been characterized by the ambition of creating a
homogenous, white Chilean citizen—a process that has been referred to
as the *blanqueo* or whitening of the population (Montecino 1996: 20).
The mestizo, considered almost white, was regarded as the prototype of
the modern Chilean and associated with advanced civilization; in contrast,
the indigenous population is today both culturally and politically marginalized and often characterized as backward, ignorant and uncivilized.[9]
Wanglen's doctor therefore represents a typical position in Chilean society
of rejecting what are perceived as indigenous values and identity.

A second olvido is the creation of social inequalities as a product of the
modern capitalist state. Inspired by the work of Tomás Moulian (1997)
and Clara Han's (2004, 2012) work on depression and state violence, I
propose that the present-day national identity and class divisions reflect an
ongoing trauma of contemporary Chile which is due to the effect of the
neo-liberal politics of the military regime of Augusto Pinochet (1973–1989).

A third olvido is the cultural repression of memories of state violence.
That is, how are stories of oppression and violence articulated and negotiated in illness experiences and medical practice? In the everyday life of
Chile today, the widespread oppression and violence of Pinochet's regime,
lasting from 1973 to 1989, are very rarely mentioned. According to historian Steve Stern (2006), many Chileans believed that the violence committed by the state during Pinochet's military dictatorship was an
impossibility, that fundamentally their society was too civilized, too law
abiding, too democratic. However, records of state violence present a different version: credible estimates claim that up to 400,000 persons were
subjected to torture during the regime (Stern 2006: xxii). During my

---

[9] This viewpoint is, in present-day Chile, especially promoted by the historian Sergio
Villalobos, who was considered the country's national historian during the military regime.
Among the practices which he associates with the Mapuche culture are polygamy, homosexu-
ality and sacrifice ("El Mercurio", May 14, 2000).

fieldwork in 2004 and 2005,[10] I often found that the record of violence had disappeared into collective oblivion, what has been referred to by Chilean academics as an olvido (Moulian 1997; Montecino 1996). Thus I also explore how the idiom of shamanistic healing practice provides the patients with a bodily outlet for expressing and negotiating experiences of violence and terror.

EMBODIMENT AND MEDICAL PLURALISM

By focusing on illness experiences, medical choices and socio-political processes, I follow a stream within medical anthropology which connects the study of illness to the notion of agency and power. This approach moves beyond meaning-based interpretations, addressing the socio-political context of illness by examining how the process of seeking recourse to medical experts (i.e. biomedical and Mapuche) affords different discursive opportunities for people to renegotiate the meaning and embodied experience of an illness within the constraints and affordances of these two medical traditions.

Two tendencies within anthropology emerged during the 1980s which became a turning point for medical anthropology: firstly, a focus on embodiment, implying a notion of the body as the "existential ground of culture" (Csordas 1988, 1994a, b, 1999, 2002); and secondly, what was labelled the critical-interpretive approach, which aimed to reconcile issues of socio-economic context and political power with the patient's subjective experience. This led to a distinction in medical anthropology between the individual, the social body and body politics (Scheper-Hughes and Lock 1987; Lock and Scheper-Hughes 1990). The body here represents the link between socio-political processes and individual experience, and what Ivo Quaranta (2001) calls the "engine of the process of inscription and projection". In consequence, illness is also ascribed a creative dimension and power due the articulation of a social order. Thus, the assumption is that the study of illness and medical practices serves as a window onto the dynamic processes through which complex identities are constituted and articulated. It is also suggested that medicine and illness are possible resources for constituting human agency, reality and identity within a broader national context. According to Miles

---

[10] Discussion of the subject, however, had recently started due to a report published in October 2003 entitled "Informe de la Comisión Verdad Histórica y Nuevo Trato". Ministerio del Interior de Chile (2003).

and Leatherman (2003), the choice of one or more forms of medicine reflects not degrees of rationality, but degrees of negotiation among myriad social forces, including the perception of the efficacy of the treatment. It has also been argued that modernity is framed in some contexts as resulting in increased choice and the enhanced rights of the individual, while it actually serves to reinforce existing political structures and power relations (Nichter and Lock 2002: 26). The existence and treatment of Mapuche illnesses in a pluralistic healing context are consequently regarded as an approach to the study of human agency in conditions of modernity: indications of how people articulate and negotiate cultural identity, social relations and power relations in a multicultural contemporary society.

Inspired by Miles and Leatherman (2003: 10), I suggest that the articulation of folk illnesses references a bodily idiom or even comprises a symbolic statement of socio-political reality, as well as a re-evaluation of cultural and national identity. Some writers have gone further to suggest that the bodily idioms of indigenous medicine, with their emphasis on traditional values, serve as a means to resist the penetration of capitalist ideology (Mysik 1998: 188). The use of traditional healing provides the patient with a diagnosis, a medicine and an idiom of suffering and affliction which profoundly affect the possibility for acting on a bodily state. In line with recent work on cosmologies and shamanism, I further suggest that indigenous cosmologies are more than merely symbolic—they are to be considered an ontology and, as such, do not only provide a language, but also a way of being and acting in the world. This corresponds with Vivieros de Castro's notion that indigenous worldviews and "animism" provide a "socio-centric" model in which categories and social relations are used to map the universe (de Castro 1998: 477).[11] As also suggested

---

[11] The ontological turn has in recent years made a valuable contribution to the study of shamanism (de Castro 2004) and materiality (Henare et al. 2007; Petersen 2011). Viviero de Castro has proposed the term "perspectivism", which inverts the Western distinction between nature (as a given) and culture (as a variable) and instead focuses on the distinctions between humans and non-humans. In the anthology *Thinking Through Things* (Henare et al. 2007), it is argued that we should take things seriously in and of themselves. It is proposed that objects and practices in different cultural and social settings should be explored not just as artefacts upon which people bestow meaning by virtue of use, but as ontologically important in their own right. The authors argue, furthermore, that we need to withdraw from the assumption that humans live in the same "world", because different people and cultural and social groups represent and understand the world in various ways. Rather, we need to acknowledge that humans inhabit not a single but numerous "worlds" and "treat meaning and thing as an identity" (Henare et al. 2007: 4). I sympathize with the approach of treating

by Petersen (2011) and Kelly (2011), medical realities are resources that people tap into and which thus contribute to forming their personhood. Moreover, drawing on Kristensen (2015), I find that the ontological is always part and parcel of relational and socio-political processes. In order to position my approach, in the next section I briefly present historical developments in respect of notions of mind, body and society within anthropology and psychiatry.

MIND AND SOCIETY

In his famous essay "The Effectiveness of Symbols", Claude Lévi-Strauss (1949) describes a shamanistic singing ritual for facilitating a difficult childbirth among the Cuna Indians in Panama. The song recited expresses the shaman's quest to capture the lost soul (*purba*) of the patient, and also, according to assumptions in the article, provides the patient with a language for expressing her psychological state and pain. This act, Lévi-Strauss argues, gives the patient an opportunity to relieve and release physical pain, because the myth provides the woman with an intellectual understanding of her pain (by providing a meaning), thereby serving to restore a sense of wellness. The healing is consequently explained through the shaman's use of myth and symbols which have the capacity to restore a sense of order by manipulating the unconscious to resolve conflicts, which in turn acts on organic processes. The effectiveness of symbols is therefore characterized as an "inductive property", whereby the unconscious mind, organic processes and rational thought act on each other.

Levi-Strauss's article can be seen as paradigmatic in two senses. Firstly, it reproduces and supports a fundamental Western body/mind dualism and the assumption that the key to healing the body is intellectual understanding, which provides a sense of wellness; in other words, the woman becomes well because she is provided with a framework of meaning which makes her believe she can get better. Hence, curing takes place through the mind. Secondly, this assumption has influenced anthropological theories of ritual and healing in which a meaning-centred approach has dominated, especially with the work of Arthur Kleinman (1986, 1994) and Mark Nichter (1981) and their use of the psychosocial model, according to which bodily distress

a medical reality as an ontology; however, I regard it as emerging from the engagement with reality, and therefore sensitive to, and part of parcel of, social and political dynamics (see Kristensen 2015).

is a product of repressed feelings. Arthur Kleinman's introduction of the concept of the "explanatory model"[12] in the 1980s, which focused on the "definition of etiology, the onset of symptoms, pathophysiology, course of sickness and treatment" in medical communication between patient and practitioner, was also informed by the meaning-centred approach (Janzen 2002: 39). The distinction between disease and illness became important, disease being regarded as the objective reality of pathology, known to any medical professional, with illness referring to its subjective dimensions. This led to the viewpoint that manifestations of depression are often somatized; that is, that patients often express psychological states through physical symptoms. Culture-bound syndromes and idioms of distress became part of this approach.

The connections outlined by Levi-Strauss, Kleinman and Nichter—between body and mind, rational thought and unconscious processes—appear rather mysterious, however, thereby raising some fundamental questions. Firstly, Levi-Strauss's article on the curing ritual fails to tell us why and how the woman perceives the medicine to be effective. This question is especially pertinent in modern fieldwork in the Latin American context, where it is almost unthinkable for a shamanistic rite to be the sole path to healing. If, under contemporary conditions, a patient prefers to consult a shaman despite biomedical doctors being regarded as the official health practitioners, what are the social implications of this preference? Furthermore, as already described in Wanglen's case, patients in the Chilean context rarely restrict themselves to one type of diagnosis but, rather, combine and move between different types of healing practices in order to treat their symptoms.

Levi-Strauss leaves another, even more crucial, question unresolved: namely, what is the link between the individual physical body and the social body or socio-political reality? This cannot be answered on the basis of his data; the article says nothing of the woman's experiences of the ritual, nor, more critically, does he offer her account and response to the question of whether she feels herself to be effectively cured. Furthermore, no indication of the social, cultural and political context beyond the scene of healing is given. This can be linked to the question of whether the articulation and experience of memory can be reduced to a single mental,

---

[12] This approach characterized Kleinman's writing in the 1980s; later he advocated an approach based on the concepts of embodiment and the socio-somatic (Kleinman 1994; Kleinman and Becker 1998).

bodily and psychosomatic function or if it is, rather, an element of complex social, cultural and political processes (Crapanzano 2004: 70). To explore this question further, in the following section I examine Freud's influence on models of the mind in psychiatry and anthropology.

FROM THE INTRAPSYCHIC TO THE PSYCHOSOCIAL MODEL

The influence of Freud and his colleagues can be traced in modern psychiatric theories of trauma and somatization, which I refer to as the intrapsychic model. Freud suggested that certain physical symptoms could be the expression of a particular intrapsychic conflict (Littlewood and Dein 2000: 14), meaning that somatic complaints can be ascribed to the repression of emotional conflicts and traumatic memories. Today, the term somatization is generally used to refer to the condition wherein mental states and experiences are expressed as bodily symptoms. Or, in the words of Henry Maudsley, "The sorrow that has no vent in tears makes other organs weep" (Littlewood and Dein 2000: 14).

Somatization as a descriptive term became widespread with its introduction in DSM III (Mai 2004: 652). It also appears in the diagnosis of post-traumatic stress disorder, one of the characteristics of which, along with the intrusive re-experiencing of elements of the trauma in nightmares and flashbacks, is somatic symptoms. If past memories are not allowed to be expressed openly, they "speak" through the body (Beneduce 2016). The bodily symptoms are manifestations of "forgotten" or "repressed" experiences and memories that are "buried" in the mind. This reflects the view of trauma as engendering amnesia and silence (Argenti and Schramm 2006). Psychiatric disorders are perceived as mental disorders, notwithstanding their prominent somatic symptoms. The medical conditions are physical, and if they cause mental symptoms these are thought of as by-products of a disturbed physiology (Kirmayer and Young 1998: 422). When health problems fall outside of these categories, physicians resort to the label of somatization. In what follows I show that this viewpoint has influenced anthropological studies, as it has been suggested that it is a dominant mode of expressing social and personal distress in non-Western societies (Kleinman 1986).

The Freudian notion that symptoms express repressed feeling that is psychological and/or psychosocial in origin—the "intrapsychic model"—became modified in medical anthropology and produced the "psychosocial model" in the study of idioms of distress (Nichter 1981). These are regarded as a way to study local illness experiences without trying to "fit" them to an appropriate biomedical disease category. In the "psychosocial model", somatization is regarded as an "important idiom through which distress is communicated": distress which is produced by role stress (Rubel et al. 1984) or "limited opportunities to ventilate feelings and seek support" due to cultural values, norms and stereotypes (Nichter 1981: 379).

A similar approach can be found in studies on depression. Some research studies (Cheung cited in Kleinman 1986) have indicated that depression and somatization are particularly common in non-Western societies and among rural, ethnic and lower-class groups. In a study in Hong Kong of depression among Chinese patients, somatic symptoms such as tiredness, fatigue, pains and gastrointestinal/cardiovascular symptoms were taken as indications of depressed mood, of which the patients were not aware, which might point to difficulties in verbalizing inner feelings (Kleinman 1986: 53); when asked directly, most of the patients admitted to feelings of sadness. The researchers concluded that, for most working-class Chinese, "conceptualization at the psychic level may seem too abstract" (Kleinman 1986: 54). Consequently, in order to explain why depressed Chinese patients have somatic symptoms, a purely psychological approach is supplemented with a cultural explanation. Kleinman points out that "culturally shaped psychological processes lead Chinese to suppress distressing emotions" (1986: 54).

Kleinman and Nichter's contributions are very valuable, as they do not assume that illness and culture-bound syndromes only take place within the individual mind, an idea that fails to integrate the dimension of culture. When the body "speaks" in somatic complaints without an obvious organic pathology, it is because the mind is not capable of expressing itself. Somatic symptoms occur because they form part of a culturally acceptable form of expressing distress. If experiences and memories are "forgotten", this is not a clinical inevitability that occurs only at the individual level; rather, it is also part of a "cultural behavioural repertoire" (Nichter 1981: 379).

CULTURE-BOUND SYNDROMES REVISITED: THE "SOCIOSOMATIC" MODEL

In anthropology, the link between culture and illness was also addressed in the study of so-called culture-bound syndromes (Yap 2001 [Chiang]). The phrase "culture-bound" gained a firm foothold in anthropology in 1985, when Simons and Hughes published their book *The Culture-Bound*

Syndromes: Folk Illnesses of Psychiatric and Anthropological Interest, which provided a framework for the development of a holistic set of descriptive characteristics of a person in a particular cultural situation; that is, the focus is on the dynamic interplay between personality functioning and socio-cultural context (1985: 3). The book debates the issue of whether these folk illnesses were in fact "authentic" medical diseases or just local manifestations of universal disease categories. A large interdisciplinary study of susto, published in 1984, concluded that the patients who were diagnosed with susto could be considered ill from a biomedical point of view, mainly suffering from infective and parasitic diseases or anaemia (Rubel et al. 1984: 87); however, no single organic syndrome or disturbance was found. The study concluded that susto could not be regarded as a syndrome or be classified as a disease in a medical sense, as the symptoms did not correspond to one diagnosis but formed a diffuse set, therefore susto was perceived as a local way of articulating and dealing with social stress; it was further clarified that many of what are known as culture-bound syndromes are in fact local ways of explaining and dealing with illness. Mark Nichter's terms "idioms of distress" and the "psychosocial model" became accepted ways of characterizing these—by Western standards—"unusual" ways of being ill.

In the mid-1980s the debate on culture-bound syndromes was intense. However, during the 1990s the study of the phenomenon almost disappeared from the anthropological literature. Several explanations might be relevant, such as the evidence that susto was not really a syndrome at all, at least not in a biomedical sense, or the fate of culture in psychiatry.[13] In

---

[13] In 1991 the National Institute of Mental Health (NIMH) recognized the special problem of diagnosis in a culturally diverse population and supported the formation of a group for culture and diagnosis, which included American anthropologists and psychiatrists. Its general goal was to suggest how to make culture more specific to DSM-IV (Lewis-Fernandéz 1996: 133). In the fourth edition of DSM, it is noted that culture-bound syndromes are "generally limited to specific societies or culture areas and are localized, folk, diagnostic categories". The manual further contains two appendices relevant for the issue of culture: (1) a cultural formulation designed to assist the clinician in evaluating and reporting the impact of the individual's cultural context; and (2) an appendix with 27 so-called culture-bound syndromes, among these some with exotic names (Lewis-Fernandéz 1996; Johansen 2006), such as ghost sickness, koro and amok. The commission felt that its serious and dedicated work towards integrating culture into the manual had been completely distorted. Kleinman dismissed the appendix as "little more than a sop thrown to cultural psychiatrists and psychiatric anthropologists" (Good 1997). These critiques led to changes in the fifth edition of DSM, which included a "Cultural Formulation Interview" (CFI) which was intended to elicit information about the socio-cultural context in which difficulties are

the wake of this development, the term "culture-bound syndromes" disappeared from anthropology and was replaced with the more neutral notion of "cultural models" (Kirmayer and Sartorius 2007). The original question addressed by the term is, however, still of relevance. In the socio-somatic model, culture-bound syndromes—in this case Mapuche ill-nesses—are linked to a social context, so that culture must be understood as associated not only with a place or community, but also with notions of heterogeneity, and social and political power relations. Hence, in the socio-somatic model the study of culture-bound syndromes or idioms of distress can serve as an approach to explore the relationship between ill-ness experience, medical practice and socio-political reality.

This argument had already been proposed in the 1980s by Libbet Crandon-Malamud when she published her work on medical pluralism and social change in Bolivia (1983, 1986, 1991, 2003). According to Crandon-Malamud, if culture-bound syndromes cannot be linked to a biomedical condition, then there must be something else going on. She proposes that the reason that people choose or accept the diagnosis of susto has to do with a negotiation of social and cultural inequalities and power relations, thereby linking it to a larger socio-political reality. However, Crandon-Malamud died before she could elaborate on her ideas, and with her, apparently, the concept of culture-bound syndromes also disappeared. Nonetheless, some of the old syndromes such as susto and nervios are treated as folk illnesses and as local idioms of distress and approached in their specific national con-text (Baer et al. 2003; Guarnaccia 1993, 2003; Low 1988; Kohrt et al. 2004). Libbet's question regarding the link between illness experience, dis-ease categories and socio-political reality seems to vanish in the focus on comparisons of different national contexts and the meaning of folk illnesses in these contexts. The tendency to treat symptoms that do not "fit" Western biomedical categories as manifestations of repressed psychological and social

experienced. In addition, the notion of culture-bound syndromes had been addressed by three concepts: (1) cultural syndromes: "clusters of symptoms and attributions that tend to co-occur among individuals in specific cultural groups, communities, or contexts ... that are recognized locally as coherent patterns of experience" (ibid.: 758); (2) cultural idioms of distress: "ways of expressing distress that may not involve specific symptoms or syndromes, but that provide collective, shared ways of experiencing and talking about personal or social concerns" (ibid.: 758); and (3) cultural explanations of distress or perceived causes: "labels, attributions, or features of an explanatory model that indicate culturally recognized mean-ing or etiology for symptoms, illness, or distress" (ibid.: 758) (see Panter-Brick and Eggerman 2017).

conflict has recently been modified in what is coined global mental health.[14] Here it is argued that illnesses are not only problems experienced by individuals, but must be understood and treated at social and cultural levels (Panter-Brick and Eggerman 2017).

From my own work, it appears that choosing between (or choosing to combine) biomedical diagnoses or folk illnesses is linked to the making of personhood and reflects the articulation and negotiation of identity and power relations. Wanglen's case of susto showed that illness experiences and medical choices are embedded in negotiations of cultural identity and political power. Furthermore, it challenged the assumption that culture-bound syndromes are purely psychological in origin. Therefore I propose—inspired by Libbet Crandon-Malamud—that, rather than exploring, for instance, what susto is in context, it is more interesting to look at the following two questions: How does the choice of this disease category by certain classes of people relate to a larger social, cultural and political context? What are the social implications of choosing a particular disease category? Furthermore, I propose to transpose the notion of trauma from an individual to a cultural and collective level. A term that is much used recently is "cultural trauma", which refers to the assumption that trauma is not the result of an individual or group experiencing pain, but is, rather, the result of discomfort entering the core of the collectivity's sense of its own identity. Collective actors "decide" (or do not decide) to represent social pain as a fundamental threat to the sense of "who they are, where they came from, and where they want to go" (Alexander et al. 2004: 10).

In his book *On Collective Memory* (1992), Maurice Halbwachs argued that there is no such thing as individual memory, and that it is only through our membership of social groups that we are able to acquire, localize and recall memories, as these groups provide the mental and material spaces necessary for the recollection of memories. A central point in this work, inspired by Halbwachs's thought, is that illness symptoms might also serve to articulate collective memories which cannot be articulated directly, which are aspects of realities connected to social and political processes. In my empirical material it appears that the illness experience and memories

---

[14]The term "global mental health" (GMH) was coined in 2001. It is a movement that consists of stakeholders advocating for equity in mental health across the globe. The emergence of GMH has been linked to developments in the field of global health, which has been defined as "the area of study, research and practice that places a priority on improving health and achieving equity in health for all people worldwide". GMH has been a target of criticism due to its biomedical domination (Patel 2012; Panter-Brick and Eggerman 2017).

"speak" of much more than individual bodily discomfort; fragments of apparently "forgotten" memories also appear, presented in metaphors and symbols that reflect socio-political reality. Therefore, my focus is on social and collective forms of forgetting rather than purely individual forms. I analyse processes that connect the physical and social bodies by focusing on social conflict as well as social forms of forgetting, the olvido, exploring olvidos as examples of the "uncanny" (Freud 1955) not in a psychoanalytic way as repressed instincts or traumatic experiences which appear in a childish fantasy, but as experiences which are influenced by socio-political processes. That is, they are experiences which, due to a collective framework within the structure of the state, are not verbalized directly, but are expressed in illness experiences and treated in medical practices as a sort of meta-reality or second-world reality (Argenti 1998, 2001).[15] Consequently, "forgetting" is not only an individual occurrence, but is also dependent on a social and collective framework for selecting experiences as well as bodily practices for the transfer of society's memory across generations (Connerton 1989).

Here I examine how a collective framework for selecting experiences worthy of recall ignores certain experiences and memories, which can, however, be allowed alternative spaces for articulation as a sort of meta-reality. Indigenous disease categories and medical practices are taken as one such alternative space. I also propose to connect Mapuche illness to the study of cultural categories and collective mechanisms for selecting memories, thereby highlighting the role that illness experiences and medical practices play in a given context. Furthermore, I highlight the importance of referential dissonance or resonance between life experience, social environment and medical practitioners. This, however, leaves unaddressed a crucial question regarding the socio-somatic model of illness experience; that is, how should we analyse the link between individual experience of illness, collective experiences and socio-political reality? This book builds on the stream of literature within medical anthropology that takes the body and embodiment as the starting point for the "making" of people, which takes place in the relation between "people who are known about, the knowledge about them, and the knowers" (Hacking 1995: 6).

---

[15] The concept of "second-world reality" is inspired by Nicolas Argenti's work on performance and violence in Cameroon's Bamenda Grassfields, where he argues that children and adults use masquerades to negotiate power relations in a meta-reality, which is useful because it relates to everyday lived reality. Therefore, he argues that the performances are not unreal in the Freudian sense as a fantasy removed from reality, but are (*sur*)real engagements with a socio-political environment.

THE BODY AND EMBODIMENT

In many works on medicine and illness, and within disciplines like anthropology, philosophy, psychology and sociology, the concepts of embodiment and the body became increasingly important during the 1990s (Csordas 1994a, b, 1999, 2002; Desjarlais 1992; Johannessen 2005; Lock 1993; Scheper-Hughes and Lock 1987; Lock and Scheper-Hughes 1990; Pizza 2005; Quaranta 2001; Scheper-Hughes 1993, 1994; Turner 1992, 1996). Embodiment is described by Thomas Csordas as "an existential condition in which the body is the subjective source or intersubjective ground of experience" (Csordas 1999: 181). The work of Csordas and that of Lock and Scheper-Hughes stand out as paradigmatic in this line of work within medical anthropology.

Csordas grounds his work in Merleau-Ponty's idea of the human body as an important object of anthropological study. He is not, however, referring to the physical human body, but the performing body or the embodied subject as the existential ground of culture and self. According to Csordas, the body becomes a "setting in relation to the world", and consciousness "the body projecting itself into the world" (Csordas 1994a: 7). Therefore, he claims, it is not legitimate to distinguish between mind and body on the level of perception. Rather, it is relevant to ask how the body *becomes* objectified through processes of reflection (Csordas 1994a: 9). That is, rather than focusing primarily on the person already objectified as a "culturally constituted *representation* of self", he wants to address the pre-objective self as a "culturally constituted mode of *being in the world*" (Csordas 1994a: 14; emphasis in original). Further, he writes that recognizing the inchoate as the existential ground of the person means that there is always some form in which the self is objectified (Csordas 1994a: 15). In order to study these processes of self-objectification, Csordas proposes a focus on language and metaphor, arguing that phenomenology and semiotics are complementary. He refers to language as a medium of intersubjectivity that gives authentic access to experience, so that language not only represents but (as Heidegger said) "discloses" (Csordas 1994a: xiii).

Nancy Scheper-Hughes and Margaret Lock's article "A Critical-Interpretive Approach in Medical Anthropology: Rituals and Routines of Discipline and Dissent" (1990) likewise aims at combining a focus on the body as experience with the body as representation. They analyse the human body as a coded metaphor and an arena for socio-political struggles. The article has become classic reading within what is referred to as "critical medical anthropology" (Janzen 2002: 42; Baer et al. 1995). It outlines an approach based on an analytical use of the body in three senses. Firstly, there is the "individual body", which refers to the phenomenological sense and experience of the bodily self (Merleau-Ponty 1962). Secondly, the article introduces the concept of "the social body". This analytical tool is based on the work of Mary Douglas (1970) and Emile Durkheim (1964), who argued that the body can be considered a natural symbol and a powerful source of metaphor. That is, they envisioned the body as a reflection of social relations and the social world, while, conversely, cultural constructions of the body are considered useful for producing and reproducing visions of society and social relations. Thirdly, the article proposes the concept of "body politics". This refers to Foucault's assumption that all medical systems are lodged in their historical context and involve relations of power and control that have structured the relationship between medical practices, practitioners of health, patients and the state. The focus is on politics (what Foucault refers to as biopolitics), which serves to regulate and control individual and social bodies and also populations, demonstrated, for instance, by the implementation of sanitary programmes (Lock and Scheper-Hughes 1990: 68).

In order to link the three bodies, I propose to regard the social body as the starting point, but not only with a notion of the social as a metaphor, but also as a lived experience which emerges through engagement with the world (Desjarlais and Throop 2011: 91). This engagement and relational context are expressed and articulated in medical dialogues and practices. Language and the use of metaphors in medical dialogue are not only a means through which people experience and come to embody categories, but also a means to the making of personhood by creatively negotiating power relations and socio-political processes. While the general arguments of the use of embodiment and the three bodies are now part of the more classical readings of medical anthropology, I here explore these in a new way, as the methodological decision to make patients the main focus, relegating medical practitioners to a secondary role, provides a thought-provoking insight into the subject. The stories of patients in a context of medical pluralism facilitate exploration of how socio-economics and ethnic identification pre-exist, and also emerge from, social practices. In other words, I here focus on the link between stories of illness, subjectivities and collective identities. As Kirmayer and Young comment, patients themselves make more or less conscious and strategic choices of disease categories in their interaction with health practitioners; they may, for instance, emphasize some symptoms and ignore others in an effort to avoid psychiatric stigmatization and gain access to the medical care they deem acceptable and appropriate (Kirmayer and Young 1998: 425). Analysed from this viewpoint, medical dialogue about illness emerges not only as a way of projecting meaning, but also as a space for action in medical practices. Furthermore, the illness itself and its cure represent a cosmology—an ontology—within a specific power structure that in this case is connected to the Chilean state. A medicine is therefore a resource through which people deal with a social reality (Crandon-Malamud 1991: 139).

In order to analyse the relationship between illness stories, medical practices and state power, I also draw upon analyses of the state and violence by Bruce Kapferer (1997, 2006), Nicolas Argenti (1998, 2001), Clara Han (2004, 2012), Ana Mariella Bacigalupo (2007, 2016a, b) and Michael Taussig (1980, 1987, 1993, 1999). In his work on sorcery in Sri Lanka, Kapferer analyses ritual practices as technologies for entering what he calls "the chaotic dynamics of human realities". He describes the state as a hierarchizing, bounding and delimiting force. State dynamics are also characterized by the control of territory and acting against threats by opponents. In the case of Sri Lanka, a consequence of this hierarchical dynamic was state violence and the killing of dissenters, who were often burnt, their bodies defaced and their personal identities erased (Kapferer 2006: 108–110). Following Kapferer and Han (2012), I analyse the negotiation of power relations in medical choices within the context of the Chilean state, as state institutions and economic precariousness are intertwined with social relations, engagement and aspirations. Indigenous medical practices provide an alternative space for the articulation of certain collective experiences within this context, one in which to manage and transform these experiences. As Taussig argues, by turning to the symbols inherent in shamanistic practice, people can reflect on their symbolic potential and hope to manage sickness and suffering (Taussig 1987); moreover, healing practices are (sur)real engagements with a socio-political environment (Argenti 1998, 2001). Or, as argued by Bacigalupo (2016b: 139), spiritual beings are historical agents; they bring knowledge and power into the bodies of shamans, who through medical practice also contribute to the making of history.

THE ORGANIZATION OF THE BOOK

One of the basic tenets of the present work is that patients make use of Mapuche medical practice in order to negotiate cultural identity and social position on several levels. Firstly, through a diagnostic process and medical dialogue about the nature of illness in the social body, patients negotiate experiences of distrust and social marginalization which colour their meetings with the public health system. By using Mapuche medicine, patients replace the social experience of being marginalized in connection to the state, due to asymmetrical power relations with medical doctors, with an experience of sharing social resources with patients from an equivalent social position. In this way, through identifying with different ethnic groups, patients come to share the same social resources and medical practice which are associated with the making of personhood. Secondly, I address the notion of effectiveness in relation to the individual body, arguing that in order to be effective, Mapuche medical practice must resonate with experiences in the individual body.

I therefore begin the analysis of my material in the next chapters by exploring how the diagnostic process and medical choices are embedded in the patients' embodiment and negotiation of categories, firstly of disease categories, thereafter the categories of ethnicity and class. The use of multiple medicines—in this case mainly biomedicine and healing practices—leads to the assumption that the body is both socially produced and constructed, and fragmented into multiple identities. I argue, however, that what might seem to be confused or splintered bodily experiences are in fact a reflection of a split in the languages that inform the socio-political reality. Here medical choices become a means to mediate, even to reconcile, the repressions and fragmentations in the experience of a current reality.

The book is structured as follows. In Chap. 2, the cultural, political and historical context is presented with a focus on the development of the Chilean state, and more specifically on issues of cultural identity, social inequalities and state violence. Chapters 3, 4, 5, 6, and 7 consist of analysis of the empirical ethnographic material. I begin by exploring diagnostic procedures and their attendant social processes, followed by analysis of how diagnosis and treatment relate to the olvidos of Chile: firstly to categories of ethnicity and class, and secondly to memory and violence. In Chap. 3, I discuss the medical practices of biomedicine and Mapuche medicine in contemporary Chile. On this background the medical gaze of the health practitioners is explored and analysed through scenes from medical practice. It is argued that the categories of disease in biomedical/psychiatric practice and in shamanistic healing practice lead to fundamentally different notions of the patient's body, which have different implications for the patient's relationship with his or her social world. In Chap. 4, cases of patients—mestizo and Mapuche—with a Mapuche illness are examined. The question here, inspired by Libbet Crandon-Malamud's (1983) article "Why Susto?", concerns the possibilities for expression of identity, agency and social positions that the diagnosis of susto offers patients. In Chap. 5, the illness stories of two Mapuche men who have migrated to the city are discussed, and their complex notions of illness, which include a number of disease categories and aetiological explanations, described. Chapter 6 investigates the connection between illness experiences and state violence in relation to the appearance of spirits in the patients' subjective experiences. Freud's concept of the uncanny is analysed, not in the original psychoanalytic sense as a part of the individual mind, but as part of a collective framework for remembering and acting in connection with experiences of terror and destruction. In Chap. 7, the focus is on the healing performance of a famous shaman (machi), José Caripan, mentioned earlier in connection with Wanglen's case. I explore how shamanistic practice provides patients with a language to express and act upon a social reality. The conclusion, discussed in detail in Chap. 8, is that indigenous medical practice provides a meta-reality for dealing with issues of identity, asymmetrical power relations and class inequalities. Ultimately, the work argues that indigenous medicine opens a space for articulation and management of collective experiences and sufferings.

References

Alexander, J., et al. 2004. *Cultural Trauma and Collective Identity.* Berkeley: University of California Press.

Antze, Paul. 1996. Telling Stories, Making Selves: Memory and Identity in Multiple Personality Disorder. In: Paul Antze & Michael Lambek (eds.), *Tense Past: Cultural Essays in Trauma and Memory.* New York: Routledge, pp. 3–25.

Argenti, Nicolas. 1998. Air Youth: Performance, Violence and the State in Cameroon. *Journal of the Royal Anthropological Institute* 4(4): 753–782.

Argenti, Nicolas. 2001. *Kesum-body* and the Places of the Gods: The Politics of Children's Masking and Second-world Realities in Oku (Cameroon). *Journal of the Royal Anthropological Institute* 7(1): 67–94.

Argenti, Nicolas & Katharina Schramm. 2006. *Violence and Memory*. Position paper presented at EASA Conference.

Bacigalupo, Ana Mariella. 2001. *La Voz del Kultrun en la Modernidad: Tradicion y Cambio en la Terapeutica de Siete Machi Mapuche*. Santiago de Chile: Ediciones Universidad Catolica de Chile.

Bacigalupo, Ana Mariella. 2007. *Thunder Shaman. Making History with Mapuche Spirits in Chile and Patagonia*. Texas: University of Texas Press.

Bacigalupo, Ana Mariella. 2016a. *Shamans of the Foye Tree. Gender, Power, and Healing among Chilean Mapuche*. Texas: University of Texas Press.

Bacigalupo, Ana Mariella. 2016b. The Paradox of Disremembering the Dead: Ritual, Memory, and Embodied Historicity in Mapuche Shamanic Personhood. *Anthropology and Humanism* 41.

Baer, Hans, Merrill Singer & Ida Susser. 1995. What is Medical Anthropology About? In: Hans Baer & Merrill Singer (eds.), *Medical Anthropology and the World System: A Critical Perspective*. Westport, Connecticut: Bergin & Garvey, pp. 1–37.

Baer, Roberta, et al. 2003. A Cross-Cultural Approach to the Study of the Folk Illness Nervios. *Culture, Medicine and Psychiatry* 27: 315–337.

Beneduce, R. 2016. Traumatic pasts and the historical imagination: symptoms of loss, postcolonial suffering, and counter-memories among African migrants. *Transcultural psychiatry*, 53(3), pp. 261–285.

Connerton, Paul. 1989. *How Societies Remember*. Cambridge: Cambridge University Press.

Crandon-Malamud, Libbet. 1983. Why Susto. *Ethnology. An International Journal of Cultural and Social Anthropology* XXII: 153–169.

Crandon-Malamud, Libbet. 1986. Medical Dialogue and the Political Economy of Medical Pluralism: a Case from Rural Highland Bolivia. *American Ethnologist* 13(3): 463–477.

Crandon-Malamud, Libbet. 1991. *From the Fat of our Souls: Social Change, Political Process, and Medical Pluralism in Bolivia*. Berkeley: University of California Press.

Crandon-Malamud, Libbet. 2003. Changing Times and Changing Symptoms: the Effects of Modernization of Mestizo Medicine in Rural Bolivia (the Case of Two Mestizo Sisters). In: Joan D. Koss-Chioino, Thomas Leatherman & Christine Greenway (eds.), *Medical Pluralism in the Andes*. Psychology Press, pp. 27–42.

Crapanzano, Vincent. 2004. *Imaginative Horizons: An Essay in Literary-philosophical Anthropology*. Chicago and London: University of Chicago Press.

Csordas, Thomas. 1988. Embodiment as a Paradigm for Anthropology. *Ethos* 18(1): 5–47. Retrieved from http://www.jstor.org/stable/640395.

Csordas, Thomas. 1994a. *The Sacred Self: A Cultural Phenomenology of Charismatic Healing*. Berkeley and Los Angeles: University of California Press.

Csordas, Thomas. 1994b. Introduction: The Body as Representation and Being-in-the-world. In: Thomas Csordas (ed.), *Embodiment and Experience: The Existential Ground of Culture and Self.* Cambridge: Cambridge University Press, pp. 1–27.

Csordas, Thomas. 1999. The Body's Career in Anthropology. In: Henrietta Moore (ed.), *Anthropological Theory Today.* Cambridge: Polity Press, pp. 193–205.

Csordas, Thomas. 2002 (1988). Embodiment as a Paradigm for Anthropology. In: *Body/Meaning/Healing.* New York: Palgrave Macmillan, pp. 58–88.

De Castro, E.V. 1998. Cosmological deixis and Amerindian perspectivism. *Journal of the Royal Anthropological Institute:* 469–488.

De Castro, E.V. 2004. Exchanging Perspectives: The Transformation of Objects into Subjects in Amerindian Ontologies. *Common Knowledge* 10(3): 463–484.

Desjarlais, R. 1992. *Body and emotion: The aesthetics of illness and healing in the Nepal Himalayas.* University of Pennsylvania Press.

Desjarlais, R. & C. Jason Throop. 2011. Phenomenological approaches in anthropology. *Annual Review of Anthropology* 40: 87–102.

Douglas, Mary. 1970. *Natural Symbols.* Middlesex: Penguin Books.

Durkheim, Emile. 1964. *The Elementary Forms of Religious Life.* London: Alden.

Freud, Sigmund. 1955 (1919). The 'Uncanny' [*Das unheimliche*]. From Standard Edition, Vol. XVII, trans. James Strachey. London: Hogarth Press, pp. 217–256.

Gluckman, M. 1958. *Analysis of a Social Situation in Modern Zululand.* The Rhodes-Livingstone papers, number twenty-eight. New York: Manchester University Press.

Gluckman, M. 2006. Ethnographic Data in British Social Anthropology. In: T.M.S. Evens & Don Handelman (eds.), *The Manchester School: Practice and Ethnographic Praxis in Anthropology.* New York and Oxford: Berghahn Books, pp. 13–25.

Good, Byron J. 1997. Studying Mental Illness in Context: Local, Global, or Universal? *Ethos* 25(2): 230–248.

Guarnaccia, Peter. 1993. Ataques de Nervios in Puerto Rico: Culture-Bound Syndromes or Popular Illness. *Medical Anthropology* 15: 157–1965.

Guarnaccia, Peter. 2003. Editorial. *Culture, Medicine and Psychiatry* 27: 249–257.

Hacking, Ian. 1995. *Rewriting the Soul: Multiple Personality and the Sciences of Memory.* Princeton, NJ: Princeton University Press.

Hacking, Ian. 1996. Memory Sciences, Memory Politics. In: Paul Antze & Michael Lambek (eds.), *Tense Past: Cultural Essays in Trauma and Memory.* New York: Routledge, pp. 67–89.

Halbwachs, Maurice. 1992. *On Collective Memory.* London: University of Chicago Press.

Han, Clara. 2004. The Work of Indebtedness: The Traumatic Present of Late Capitalist Chile. *Culture, Medicine and Psychiatry* 28(2): 169–187.

Han, Clara. 2012. *Life in Debt. Times of Care and Violence in Neoliberal Chile.* London: University of California Press.

Henare, Amiria, Martin Holbraad & Sari Wastell. 2007. Introduction. In: A. Henare, M. Holbraad & S. Wastell (eds.), *Thinking through Things: Theorising Artefact Ethnographically.* London: Routledge, pp. 1–32.

Janzen, John. 1978. *The Quest for Therapy: Medical Pluralism in Lower Zaire.* Berkeley, Los Angeles, and London: University of California Press.

Janzen, John. 2002. *The Social Fabric of Health: An Introduction to Medical Anthropology.* New York: McGraw-Hill.

Johannessen, Helle. 2005. Body and Self in Medical Pluralism. In: Helle Johanessen & Imre Lázár (eds.), *Multiple Medical Realities: Patients and Healers in Biomedical, Alternative and Traditional Medicine.* Oxford and New York: Berghahn, pp. 1–21.

Johansen, Katrine Schepelern. 2006. *Kultur og Psykiatri: En Antropologi om Transkulturel Psykiatri på Danske Hospitaler.* Ph.D.- afhandling. København: Institut for Antropologi og Sct. Hans Hospital.

Kaiser, B.N., E.E. Haroz, B.A. Kohrt, P.A. Bolton, J.K. Bass & D.E. Hinton 2015. "Thinking too much": A systematic review of a common idiom of distress. *Social Science & Medicine* 147: 170–183.

Kapferer, Bruce. 1987. The Anthropology of Max Gluckman. *Social Analysis* 22: 3–21.

Kapferer, Bruce. 1997. *The Feast of the Sorcerer. Practices of Consciousness and Power.* Chicago: Chicago University Press.

Kapferer, Bruce. 2003. Sorcery, Modernity and the Constitutive Imaginary: Hybridising Continuities. In: Bruce Kapferer (ed.), *Beyond Rationalism: Rethinking Magic, Witchcraft and Sorcery.* London and New York: Berghahn Books, pp. 105–128.

Kapferer, Bruce. 2006. Situations, Crisis, and the Anthropology of the Concrete: The Contribution of Max Gluckman. In: T.M.S. & Don Handelman (eds.), *The Manchester School: Practice and Ethnographic Praxis in Anthropology.* Oxford and New York, pp. 118–159.

Kelly, José Antonio. 2011. *State Healthcare and Yanomamo Transformation. A symmetrical Ethnography:* Tucson: University of Arizona Press.

Kempny, Marian. 2006. History of the Manchester "School" and the Extended-Case Method. *Social Analysis* 49(3): 144–165.

Kirmayer, Lawrence. 2004. Explaining Medically Unexplained Symptoms. *Canadian Journal of Psychiatry* 49(10): 663–672.

Kirmayer, Lawrence & Allan Young. 1998. Culture and Somatization: Clinical, Epidemiological, and Ethnographic Perspective. *Psychosomatic Medicine* 60(4): 420–431.

Kirmayer, Lawrence & Noman Sartorius. 2007. Cultural Models and Somatic Syndromes. *Psychosomatic Medicine* 69: 832–840.

Kleinman, Arthur. 1986. *Social Origins of Distress and Disease: Depression, Neurasthenia, and Pain in Modern China.* New Haven: Yale University Press.

Kleinman, Arthur. 1994. How Bodies Remember: Social Memory and Bodily Experience of Criticism, Resistance and Delegitimation following China's Cultural Revolution. *New Literary History* 25(3), 25th Anniversary Issue: 707–723.

Kleinman, Arthur & Anne E. Becker. 1998. "Sociosomatics": The Contributions of Anthropology to Psychosomatic Medicine. *Journal of the American Psychosomatic Society* 60(4): 389–394.

Kohrt, B.A., D.J. Hruschka, H.E. Kohrt, N.L. Panebianco & G. Tsagaankhuu 2004. Distribution of distress in post-socialist Mongolia: a cultural epidemiology of yadargaa. *Social Science & Medicine* 58(3): 471–485.

Kristensen Benedikte, Møller. 2015. *Returning to the Forest: Shamanism, Landscape and History among the Duha of Northern Mongolia*. PhD thesis University of Copenhagen.

Lévi-Strauss, Claude. 2000 (1949). The Effectiveness of Symbols. In: Roland Littlewood & Simon Dein (eds.), *Cultural Psychiatry and Medical Anthropology: An Introduction and Reader*. London and New Brunswick: The Athlone Press, pp. 162–177.

Lewis-Fernandéz, R. 1996. Cultural Formulation of Psychiatric Diagnosis: Introduction. *Culture, Medicine and Psychiatry* 20: 133–144.

Littlewood, Roland & Simon Dein (eds.). 2000. Introduction. In: Roland Littlewood & Simon Dein (eds.), *Cultural Psychiatry and Medical Anthropology: An Introduction and Reader*. London and New Brunswick: The Athlone Press, pp. 1–34.

Lock, Margaret. 1993. Cultivating the Body: Anthropological and Epistemologies of Bodily Practices and Knowledge. *Annual Review of Anthropology*. 1993: 133–155.

Lock, Margaret & Nancy Scheper-Hughes. 1990. A Critical-Interpretive Approach in Medical Anthropology: Rituals and Routines of Discipline and Dissent. In: Thomas M. Johnson and Carolyn Fishel Sargent (eds.), *Medical Anthropology, Contemporary Theory and Method*. Westport: Praeger Publishers, pp. 47–73.

Lock, Margaret & Nancy Scheper-Hughes. 1996. A Critical-Interpretive Approach in Medical Anthropology: Rituals and Routines of Discipline and Dissent. In: Carolyn Fishel Sargent and Thomas M. Johnson (eds.), *Medical Anthropology, Contemporary Theory and Method*. Westport: Praeger Publishers, Rev. ed., pp. 41–70.

Low, Setha. 1988. Medical Practice in Response to a Folk Illness: The Diagnosis and Treatment of *Nervios* in Costa Rica. In: M. Lock & D.R. Gordon (eds.), *Biomedicine Examined*. Dordrecht: Kluwer Academic Publishers, 415–438.

Mai, F. 2004. Somatization disorder: a practical review. *The Canadian Journal of Psychiatry* 49(10): 652–662.

Marcus, George. 1995. Ethnography in/Of the World System: The Emergence of Multi-Sited Ethnography. *Annual Reviews* 24: 95–117.

Merleau-Ponty, Maurice. 1962. *Phenomenology of Perception*. London and New York: Routledge.

Miles, Ann & Thomas Leatherman. 2003. Perspectives on Medical Anthropology in the Andes. In: Joan D. Koss-Chioino, Thomas Leatherman & Christine Greenway (eds.), *Medical Pluralism in the Andes*. Psychology Press, pp. 3–16.

Ministerio del Interior de Chile. 2003. Decreto n.° 19: Comisión Verdad y Nuevo Trato, *Biblioteca del Congreso Nacional de Chile*.

Montecino, Sonia. 1996. *Madres y Huachos: Alegorías del Mestizaje Chileno*. Santiago: Biblioteca Claves de Chile. Editorial Sudamericana.

Moulian, Tomás. 1997. *Anatomía de un Mito*. Arcis Universidad: LOM Ediciones, Serie Punto de Fga. Coleccion sin Norte.

Mysik, Avis. 1998. Susto: An Illness of the Poor. *Dialectical Anthropology* 23: 187–202.

Nichter, Mark. 1981. Idioms of Distress: Alternatives in the Expression of Psychosocial Distress: A Case Study from South India. *Culture, Medicine and Psychiatry* 5: 379–408.

Nichter, Mark & Margaret Lock (eds.). 2002. Introduction: from Documenting Medical Pluralism to Critical Interpretations of Globalized Health Knowledge, Policies and Practices. In: Mark Nichter & Margaret Lock (eds.), *New Horizons in Medical Anthropology*, pp. 1–35.

Panter-Brick, C. & Eggerman, M. 2017. *Anthropology and Global Mental Health: Depth, Breadth, and Relevance*. In: White R., Jain S., Orr D. & Read U. (eds.), *The Palgrave Handbook of Sociocultural Perspectives on Global Mental Health*. London: Palgrave Macmillan.

Patel, V. 2012. Global mental health: from science to action. *Harvard Review of Psychiatry* 20(1): 6–12.

Petersen, Morten Axel. 2011. *Not quite Shamans. Spirit Worlds and Political Lives in Northern Mongolia*. New York: Cornell Press.

Pizza, Giovianni. 2005. *Saperi, partiche e politiche del corpo*. Roma: Carocci.

Quaranta, Ivo. 2001. Contextualising the Body: Anthropology, Biomedicine and Medical Anthropology. *Rivista Della Società Italiana Di Antropología Medica* 11–12: 155–171.

Rubel, Arthur, O'Nell Carl & Rolando Collado-Ardón. 1984. *Susto: A Folk Illness*. Berkeley and Los Angeles: University of California Press.

Scheper-Hughes, N. 1993. *Death without weeping: The violence of everyday life in Brazil*. Berkeley: University of California Press.

Scheper-Hughes, N. 1994. Embodied Knowledge: Thinking with the Body in Critical Medical Anthropology. In: Robert Borofsky (ed.), *Assessing Cultural Anthropology*. New York: McGraw-Hill, pp. 229–241.

Scheper-Hughes, Nancy & Margaret Lock. 1987. The Mindful Body: A Prolegomenon to Future Work in Medical Anthropology. *Medical Anthropology Quarterly* 1(1): 6–41.

Simons, Ronald & Charles Hughes (eds.). 1985. *The Culture-Bound Syndromes: Folk Illnesses of Psychiatric and Anthropological Interest.* Dordrecth: D. Reidel Publishing Company.

Stern, Steve. 2006. *Remembering Pinochet's Chile: On the Eve of London 1998.* Book One of the Trilogy: The Memory Box of Pinochet's Chile. Durham: Duke University Press.

Taussig, Michael. 1980. *The Devil and Commodity Fetishism in South America.* Chapel Hill: The University of North Carolina Press.

Taussig, Michael. 1987. *Shamanism, Colonialism and the Wild Man.* Chicago and London: The University of Chicago Press.

Taussig, Michael. 1993. *Mimesis and Alterity. A Particular History of the Senses.* New York: Routledge.

Taussig, Michael. 1999. *Defacement. Public Secrecy and the Labor of the Negative.* Stanford: Sanford University Press.

Turner, Brian. 1992. *Regulating Bodies: Essays in Medical Sociology.* London and New York: Routledge.

Turner, Brian. 1996. *The Body and Society: Explorations in Social Theory.* London: Sage Publications.

Turner, Victor. 1957. *Schism and Continuity in an African Society: A Study of Ndembu Village Life.* Manchester: Manchester University Press.

Turner, Victor. 1967. *Forest of Symbols: Aspects of Ndembu Ritual.* Ithaca, NY: Cornell University Press.

Van Velsen, J. 1967. The Extended-case Method and Situational Analysis. In: A.L. Epstein (ed.), *The Craft of Social Anthropology.* London: Tavistock, pp. 129–149.

Yap, P.M. 2001 (1951). Mental Diseases Peculiar to Certain Culture: a Survey of Comparative Psychiatry. In: Roland Littlewood & Simon Dein (eds.), *Cultural Psychiatry and Medical Anthropology: An Introduction and Reader.* London and New Brunswick: The Athlone Press, pp. 179–198.

CHAPTER 2

The History, Culture and Politics of Chile

The Chilean case reflects a general process of colonization followed by
modernization in Latin America, which began with Columbus's discovery
of America in 1492. New ethnic identities emerged as a consequence of
colonization, in this case the mestizo (from the Latin *mixtus*), a term which
refers to those whose biological origin is the product of racial mixture. In
a Latin American context, mestizaje refers to the process of racial mixing
between African, European and indigenous peoples. Since the late nine-
teenth century, mestizaje has played a central role in the official ideology of
Latin American national identities as the cultural and ethnic foundation of
the new nation-states. The ideology, also referred to as hybridization and
creolization,[1] was officially based on the notion of cultural mixing as har-
monious homogeneity. This has been characterized as a postmodern, postcolonial and democratic kind of politics and a source of cultural creativity
(Canclini 1989). However, as pointed out by a number of scholars, the
ideology of the mestizaje in fact obfuscated the prevalent notions of white
supremacy and the ideal of a "whitening" (*blanqueamiento*) of the population (Rahier 2003: 41; Richards 2013: 42). In the ideology of the modern
Chilean state, "indigenous" is associated with adjectives such as backward
and non-civilized, in contrast to dominant notions of a modern Chile.
According to the official history, indigenous traits are today associated with

---

[1] The term "creole" refers to a person with European blood, born outside Europe. In this
ethnic category the indigenous blood is denied (Anderson 1983: 58).

© The Author(s) 2019
D. B. Kristensen, *Patients, Doctors and Healers*,
https://doi.org/10.1007/978-3-319-97031-8_2

a heroic past resisting the colonizers, but are not, however, considered part of the modern nation.

The case of Southern Chile thereby replicates the general pattern of the process of mestizaje and modernity in Latin America, with a Spanish-speaking population designated as mestizo along with smaller indigenous minorities. Southern Chile also, however, occupies a unique position since, unlike other parts of Latin America, the national integration of the indigenous population did not take place during the initial process of colonization. Instead, as noted in the previous chapter, the native population retained autonomy in the south of Chile until 1884. Thus, today's Chile is a historical phenomenon and the result of a bloody colonial past where the colonizers sought to conquer and "whiten" the population, and in this process were influenced and "coloured" by the practices of the natives; the mestizo, for example, was the product of a sexual relationship between an indigenous woman and the European colonizer. In the nation-building of modern Chilean society, mestizaje has been shorn of its negative associations and is, rather, associated with a modern, civilized, ethnically homogenous and "white" nation. In a political sense Chile is also an extreme example of modernity, as the political model introduced by the military junta led by Augusto Pinochet (1973–1989) aimed at erasing any cultural and political activity that could threaten the neo-liberal model.

In this chapter I present the cultural and political context of present-day Chile, identifying themes of cultural and political repression. This is followed by discussion of the neo-liberal model and politics of the military regime, and the position of the Mapuche in post-dictatorship Chile. Supported by the work of Clara Han (2004, 2012), Patricia Richards (2013) and Tomás Moulian (1997), I suggest that the ideology of the military regime was based on a collective repression, violence and for-getting of cultural and social inequalities. I here present three types of olvidos: firstly, as described above, the whitening through the process of mestizaje, where indigenous roots are suppressed and denied; secondly, the theme of the social inequalities and class division produced by the integration of the Mapuche into the Chilean nation and later the intro-duction of the neo-liberal model; and thirdly, the theme of the state violence that is inflicted on the opponents of state politics, a theme that runs through the history of both colonization and later the military regime.

SPANISH COLONIZERS, MISSIONARIES AND THE INDIGENOUS POPULATION

Chilean history is based on the territorial resistance of the Mapuche to the colonizers, first the Incas and later the Spaniards. The area which is now Chile formed part of an ancestral territory called *wall mapu* or *país* Mapuche, lying between the River Copiapó in the north and Chiloé Island in the south and populated by different groups of indigenous people, including the Nagche, Wenteche, Puelche and Lafkenche, who all spoke Mapudungun (Marimán 2006: 52, 77). Chile was invaded in 1540 by the Spanish conquistador Pedro de Valdivia, who defeated substantial indigenous opposition to found the city of Santiago and the first hospitals (Jones 1999: 144). In his letters home he describes his fascination with the Chilean landscape as well as his attempt to conquer the local population, whom he and his fellows regarded as enemies of Christ and God. These letters also describe the extreme violence through which the process of colonization took place; in addition to killing thousands of Indians, de Valdivia also ordered the amputation of the hands and noses of an additional 1500–2000 (letter dated 15 October 1550, cited in Foerster 1993: 19). Later, as part of the indigenous resistance to colonization, de Valdivia was killed[2] by the Mapuche chief Lautaro[3] and all the symbols of Spanish colonization—fortresses, hospitals and missions—were destroyed. Subsequently, both soldiers and missionaries were forced to flee from the southern part of Chile (Citarella et al. 1995: 421). The Spanish army repeated its attempt to con-

[2] The killing of Pedro de Valdivia is described in detail by various chroniclers and is today very vivid in the oral memories of the Mapuche. Valdivia was captured after a Mapuche victory over the Spaniards in Tucapel and brought to Caupalican, the "Mapuche governor", following which there was a discussion of whether Valdivia should be killed immediately or spared. Valdivia pitifully asked for forgiveness (Gonzalez Galvez 2012). In one version an Indian, seeing that Caupalican was inclined to forgive Valdivia, gave Valdivia a huge blow to the head with his club (de Ercilla 1982: 165; de Ovalle 2003; Rosales 1989). According to another version, the Mapuche lit a fire nearby to Valdivia and slowly tore off pieces of his arms with shell knives, cooking and eating the flesh in front of him (Gonzalez Galvez 2012). In yet another version, the Indians wanted to punish Valdivia for his greed, and forced him to eat molten gold. After his death they made trumpets out of the bones of his legs, keeping the skull as a memento (de Ovalle 2003: 290).

[3] Alonso Ercilla was a poet employed by the Spanish crown to describe life in the Spanish colonies. He stayed 17 months in Chile, from 1557 to 1558. The Mapuche heroes, indigenous chiefs from the wars of resistance—Lautaro, Galvarino and Caupalican—are celebrated in his book *La Araucania*, which is acknowledged as the official national history, is considered national heritage and is obligatory reading in primary schools.

quer the south, but was forced to retreat due to fierce resistance by the indigenous population.[4]

According to historian José Bengoa, the indigenous population of Chile was around one million at the time of the arrival of the Spanish colonizers. By 1564 around 400,000 had died as a result of war, harsh labour systems and epidemics such as smallpox, plague, syphilis, typhus and measles (Bengoa 1985: 30; Jones 1999: 144). Despite the serious decline in the indigenous population, in 1641 the Spaniards gave up the ambition of conquering the south (beyond the River Bío Bío), although in 1673 Father Diego de Rosales asked how it was that Spain, which had been able to conquer the Aztec and Inca Empires, had been beaten by naked Mapuche with wooden weapons (Rosales 1989: 114; Bacigalupo 2007: 116).

The Mapuche were hunters and horticulturalists; they collected berries and cones and had a few crops that they supplemented with fishing, hunting and domestic herds of guanaco (*chiliweke*) (de Moesbach and Coña 2000 [1930]: 119; Bengoa 1985: 19–20). They were socio-politically structured through lineage-based marriage alliances in a kin system known as *aillarewe* (Mallon 2005: 7); although politically decentralized, this arrangement had helped to control the vast territory of *país* Mapuche and lent them the strength to resist colonization (Mariman 2006; Crow 2013: 201). They were organized in small, endogamous, patrilineal kin groups, with a local lineage head, the *lonko*, in charge of each group, which turned the confrontations between the Mapuche and colonizers into guerrilla warfare that ultimately destroyed encroaching Spanish settlements (Bacigalupo 2007: 116). Finally, in the so-called Paces de Quilín[5] (Quilín Peace), the Spanish crown recognized the southern part of the country as an independent Mapuche nation (Mariman 2006: 78; Bengoa 1985: 33; Foerster 1996: 186–187). Some Spanish soldiers remained in the area in fortresses, however, and gradually the Spanish missionaries—first the Jesuits and later the Franciscans—were permitted to return. In the case of the

---

[4] In one of the first historical documents from this period, the Spanish soldier Alonso Gonzáles de Nájera, who lived among the Auraucanians from 1606 to 1608, describes the relationship between natives and colonizers. His testimonies include the bloody description of how the indigenous crucified those they captured and hanged them from a tree; thereafter they took pieces of meat from the victims and roasted the body; lastly, they opened the chest of their victims and took out the heart (de Nájera 1971: 58–69).

[5] This event has a huge symbolic importance for the Mapuche movement today, as it points to the illegality of the Chileans' invasion of the Mapuche territory (Foerster 2001: 1, in Di Giminiani 2012: 57).

Jesuits, their critique of the Spanish colonizers' brutality helped them to gain the confidence of the indigenous population (Foerster 1996: 260, 1993: 20).

There are relatively few sources describing relations between the Mapuche and early colonizers. According to Dufey (in Caniuqueo 2006), the latter viewed the Mapuche as wild and primitive; in a letter home one "colono" described the native population as "lazy and distrustful", but also talked about friendships between the children of the two groups. In a Swiss report it was noted that "the immigrants maintain very good relations with the Mapuche that still inhabit the district" (ibid.: 155). Other historical missionary documents (Luis de Valdivia 1621; Diego de Rosales 1989; Alonso de Ovalle 2003) describe the relationship between the missionaries and the indigenous population in the southern part of Chile as one based on relative peace, mutual interest and dependency. It should be noted that these observations were all made by colonos, and do not necessarily reflect Mapuche experiences (Richards 2013: 42).

The period of Mapuche independence from the Chilean Republic was characterized by an abundance of land and livestock (Di Giminiani 2012: 55; Guevara 1913), while the native population exhibited a cultural openness to the goods, technologies and practices of the Spaniards. Many sources report lively trade between the Spaniards and the indigenous population; the natives provided salt, ponchos, cattle and horses, which they exchanged for goods, axes, swords and alcohol (Bengoa 1985: 212).[6] At the end of the sixteenth century missionaries observed that cultivating crops like corn, potatoes and beans had become a feature of Mapuche agricultural practices. Furthermore, they observed the presence of sheep, horses, apple trees and cider, which the indigenous named *muday* (Jones 1999: 147–148).

THE NATIONAL INTEGRATION OF THE INDIGENOUS POPULATION

In 1810, under the leadership of Bernardo O'Higgens, a small group of creoles declared independence from Spain; this was followed by a period of war until, in 1818, an independent Republic of Chile became a reality (Boccara and Seguel-Boccara 1999). The first decades following Chilean independence were relatively peaceful, however, as the creole leaders

---

[6] In addition, the Mapuche adopted animals that the Spanish had brought such as sheep, goats, horses and cows, as both a source of nutrition and a trading commodity (Bengoa 1985: 20).

regarded the Mapuche nation in the south as a frontier with which it was necessary to maintain peace and political union (Pinto 2000: 78); trade between colonos and the Mapuche persisted (Bengoa 1985). In the national ideology of the founding of the Chilean nation-state, indigenous peoples were depicted as heroic due to their resistance against the Spanish colonizers. Increasingly, nevertheless, the ambition to conquer the south grew in fervour and the Mapuche began to be presented as "an inferior race", as lacking in intellect and morality and a stain on the nation; their culture was characterized as uncivilized and barbaric (Jones 1999; Richards 2013; Caniuqueo 2006). The prominent nineteenth-century historian Diego Barros Arana, famous for his 16-volume *Historia general de Chile*, argued, for instance, that as a result of their barbarity the Mapuche were not capable of exploiting their land (Arana 1884, 1934).[7] His vision resonates with stereotypes of today, as he considered the Mapuche to be reserved, distrustful and drunken. In a similar vein, the politician and historian Benjamin Vicuña Mackenna denied the existence of Mapuche roots to the Chilean nation, observing, "Our People do not descend from the barbarian of Arauco, who has never wanted to submit himself to the foreigner nor ally with him". Therefore, integration and assimilation of the indigenous territory began to be regarded as fundamental to the creation of a modern nation (Richards 2013: 37–38).

The first strategy of occupation was initiated in 1861 (Di Giminiani 2012). However, as noted in the previous chapter, attempts by the Chilean army to colonize the south did not succeed until a final war lasting from 1881 to 1884, which is ironically referred to as "the pacification". The nature of this war is still ideologically disputed, as records of violence have been officially denied. Sergio Villalobos,[8] one of Chile's most recognized

---

[7] The historian Barros Arana is considered the ideological figure behind the integration of the indigenous population into the Chilean nation-state. In his works, which include *Origines de Chile: La Fundamentación de la Nacionalidad* (1934), he describes the ethnic character of the Mapuche by referring to historical documents from the period of intense war, for instance the work of the Spanish soldier Najera. Thus he completely dismisses the historical documents of the missionaries, which presented a much more peaceful and positive description of the indigenous population, as well as the relationship between the natives and the colonizers.

[8] In September 2008 in an interview in *El Mercurio*, Villalobos restated this argument as follows: "There are not exactly indigenous peoples, but rather simply mestizo groupings that formed on the old ethnic groups that existed in the country; there are mestizo descendants of the Araucanos of the Araucania. In Chile completely pure indigenous people don't exist. … The original peoples in Chile disappeared. The peoples there are now are not the origi-

historians whose books were school texts for decades, describes the integration of the Mapuche as a peaceful and natural process that only required "*Mucho mosto and mucha música*" (lots of alcohol and music; Crow 2013: 28; Richards 2013: 50), thereby, as argued by Richards, resurrecting the myth of mestizaje (Richards 2013: 50).

In contrast, historian José Bengoa, in his book *Historia de Chile* (1985), argues that this was indeed a bloody war, which he bases on oral testimonies, telegrams and newspaper articles. Joanna Crow talks about "violent raids" carried out by the Araucanians against the Chileans and, in retaliation, the assassination of "friendly Indians" by Chileans (2013: 31). Lincoqueo writes that 85% of the indigenous population was exterminated (2002). In a similar vein, Mapuche Reynaldo Mariqueo characterizes the period in the following way:

> Under the pretext of 'civilising' and 'integrating' they declared merciless war on us; their methods fully excelled those of their Spanish predecessors in their cruelty and barbarity ... Our land witnessed some of the most abominable crimes in the history of America and the world. The armies burned houses and crops; they executed captives and seized any people they found; they murdered old people, women and children and took animals and valuable objects as war booty. (Mariqueo 1989: 107)[9]

In the period following the pacification of the south, the Chilean state confiscated the territories of the Mapuche, the majority of which were sold to European settlers[10] in an attempt to civilize and "whiten" the Chilean population. This was based on the assumption that the mixing of blood from the "white race" (the Europeans) was essential to improve the Chilean race and to create a civilized nation (Boccara and Seguel-Boccara 1999). In what was referred to as a generous gesture by the Chilean government, the indigenous population was assigned an area of 500,000 hectares in the Mapuche heartland. This area was divided into collective reservations

nals, but rather their descendants." In this way Villalobos denies the continuity of indigenousness (Richards 2013: 50).

[9] During my fieldwork I also heard many oral testimonies from this period that had been suppressed; these mostly refer to the Chileans cutting off the body parts of the native population, including arms and female breasts.

[10] A European immigrant was normally granted 50–500 hectares of land (Collier 1996: 95–95).

(*comunidades*) and guaranteed to the indigenous peoples with an official document, the so-called Titulos de Merced.

Following the "pacification", the Mapuche continuously lost territory and therefore also increasingly left their traditional lifestyle behind. Between 1884 and 1927 around 3000 reservations were created in Southern Chile.[11] While before national integration the indigenous populations were, by and large, semi-nomads living on extensive agriculture and trade with the Spaniards, they were now forced to become settled farmers, even though they lacked the background to make best use of their land (Mallon 2005; Crow 2013: 47). To add to this, a serious threat to their fragile existence as farmers came in several subsequent steps. The first threat came with the law (Law Decree no. 4.169) that, in 1927, divided indigenous land into individual plots, which made the sale of this land possible (Aylwin 2000). In the following period, from 1931 to 1971, 832 of almost 3000 communities were divided, and around a fifth of the plots were sold to non-indigenous settlers (Aylwin 2002 in Richards 2013: 42). An analogy that spread in the 1940s was that Mapuche communities comprised a "suicide belt" due to the belief that the land was in "lazy hands" as "work and progress did not flourish" (Richards 2013: 57). Foerster and Montecino have argued that the use of the term suicide as opposed to "assassination" was important, as it was based on the assumption that colonos and Chileans were killing themselves by allowing the Mapuche to have land (Foerster and Montecino 1988: 278; Richards 2013: 57; Caniuqueo 2006: 180).

The advent of Salvador Allende's government (1970–1973) marked a significant change in Mapuche prospects, as the process of loss of land was reversed in an agrarian reform that returned around 100,000 hectares to Mapuche communities (Boccara and Seguel-Boccara 1999). The Mapuche in many cases comprised part of a broad front of rural poor in the leftist Popular Unity Coalition (Mallon 2005: 88). Even though Allende did not specifically address issues of Mapuche identity, instead including these people in the category of peasants, many communities experienced a new era of prosperity (Mallon 2005). This was a very short-lived development, however, and another serious blow against the Mapuche as farmers took place during the military regime of Augusto Pinochet.

---

[11] According to Boccara and Seguel-Boccara, there were 2919 Titulus de Merced, which allocated rights to 526,285 hectares of land to a total of 83,170 persons (1999: 757).

CREATING A NEW CHILE, CREATING INEQUALITY: THE NEO-LIBERAL MODEL

On 11 September 1973, Augusto Pinochet seized political and economic power in a military coup. The proclaimed goal of the military junta led by Pinochet was the imposition of a new social and political order upon Chile; a further aim was to depoliticize the country and implant the free market. To this end it initiated what it called a "modernization" and "cleansing" (*depuración*) of Chilean politics (Loveman 2001: 263). In order to arrive at a political and economic transformation of Chile, the military junta announced, in the "Declaration of Principles of the Government of Chile" (1974), its intention to "take upon itself the historic mission of giving Chile new governmental institutions that [would] embody the profound changes occurring in modern times" (ibid.: 264) Later the Declaration of Principles stressed the importance of the task of "reorganizing the economy, destroyed to its very roots by Marxism" and "imposing authority and discipline in production and labour relations". The new political system involved a strengthening of presidential authority as a "rationalized, modern, and functional public administration purified of all political and party influence" (cited in Loveman 2001: 264–265). Furthermore, the notion of the freedom of the individual was advocated as fundamental. The following extract from Constitutional Act number 3 illustrates the official ideology of the Chilean neo-liberal state during the military regime:

> Article 1: Men are born free and equal in dignity. This constitutional act guarantees all individuals.
>
> 11. Liberty of conscience, and expressions of all creeds and free exercise of all religions, as do not violate moral principles, good behaviour or public order …
>
> 12. Freedom of opinion and information, in all ways and by all means, without prior censorship, notwithstanding responsibility under the law for offence or abuse as may be committed in use of all freedom. However, the courts may prohibit publication or circulation of opinions or information affecting moral principles, public order, national security or the private life of individuals. … (cited in Loveman 2001: 271)

As a means to arrive at its political goal, the military junta dissolved congress and outlawed political parties and labour unions. A strict nighttime curfew was introduced along with a rigorous censoring of all media. Leadership of virtually all important national institutions was assigned to persons with military rank. Furthermore, all political opponents were persecuted, some through routine harassment, while others (around

7000) were herded into the national stadium in Santiago, the main centre for interrogation and torture (Collier and Sater 2004: 359–361;
Borzutsky and Oppenheim 2006: xv). To "disappear" became the destiny of a large number of opponents, particularly those with left-wing
leanings, and most of those who "disappeared" (*Lo desaparecieron*) were
never seen again (Loveman 2001: 264).

The ideological foundation for Pinochet's economic programme was
developed by "los Chicago Boys", Chilean economists who had received
their training in the Department of Economics at the University of Chicago.
In March 1975, the American professor Milton Friedman visited Chile and
talked to Pinochet about the need for "shock treatment" to eliminate infla-
tion. In April 1975, after hearing the discussion of economists at a weekend
conference, Pinochet decided to give the Chicago boys the authority to
mastermind the economic deconstruction of Chile. The primary aim was to
reverse the state-interventionist trend that had developed in Chile since the
1920s, which they accused of holding back economic growth. Furthermore,
they developed a programme for the implementation of a free market and
the privatization of social security, named "the seven modernizations",
which included changes in the areas of health, education, labour, public
administration and the judicial system (Collier and Sater 2004: 365;
Loveman 2001: 265; Paley 2001: 8). Subsequently, more than 400 state-
owned, state-controlled companies were privatized. Later, in 1980, by Law
Decrees No. 3500 and No. 3501, the privatization of social security took
place. The aim was to avoid distributing resources along class lines, and to
introduce economic incentives to undermine the capacity of collective
action by the working class (Schamis 2002: 77–78).

The privatization spurred by the military regime during the 1970s provided excellent opportunities to build up large business empires.
Construction boomed as well as consumerism, the latter strongly supported by the introduction of credit cards. In 1979 Chile's first credit card
("Diners Club de Chile") appeared, along with foreign goods including
Japanese TVs and radios, Korean automobiles (the number of cars in Chile
tripled between 1975 and 1985), French perfume and Scotch whisky. All
of this created an impression of a new, prosperous Chile. In 1980 the
Chilean government declared:

> Five years ago Chile boldly embarked on a course to revitalize its weakening
> economy, replacing protectionism with free-market politics. The average
> GDP growth rate over the last year has been 7.3%. A diversified economy

capable of functioning at an internationally competitive level has now been established, thereby assuring economic stability and offering excellent opportunities for domestic and foreign investors. (Cited in Loveman 2001: 279)

It is no wonder that the neo-liberal model implemented during this period has been called an economic miracle, with high growth accompanied by economic stability, although dissident intellectuals, artists and writers were producing work which focused on its human cost (Loveman 2001: 279). Backstage, the number of poor Chileans without any social security grew rapidly. Many from the lower strata (in 1980 about one-third of the working population) survived in "informal" occupations such as street-vending and domestic service. As a result, the informal and service sectors flourished, mainly due to the labour of poor women. In the same period the prevalence of alcoholism increased, as well as participation in evangelical churches (mainly Pentecostal): in the mid-1980s 20% of Chileans were members of an evangelical church (Collier and Sater 2004: 374).

The politics of the military regime also influenced the way of life of the indigenous population. During the government of Salvador Allende, the process of privatization of indigenous territories came to a halt when, in 1970, Law Decree no. 17,729 guaranteed the indigenous population collective rights to their territory. During the military regime this process was reversed and collective indigenous rights were abolished; in 1979 Law Decree no. 2568 stated that "the divided lands will no longer be considered indigenous lands, and the people living on those lands will no longer be considered indigenous" (Boccara 2002: 286). A minister from that epoch formulated the now-famous politics of the military regime: "In Chile there are no indigenous, only Chilean."[12] Much of the land that had been returned to the Mapuche under the agrarian reform of Salvador Allende was handed over to private owners and multinational logging companies with the aim of stimulating economic growth. The law resulted in the division of 1839 Mapuche communities between 1979 and 1982. During this time the indigenous population lost around 300,000 hectares of land (Aylwin 2000: 3), or about 40% of the land under Titulus Merced (Richards 2013: 59). In addition to the loss of land, the Mapuche became targets of the systematic oppression of Pinochet's regime, as many had joined social and political movements associated with the Unidad Popular of Salvador Allende;

[12] This was declared by the Minister of Agriculture in the "Diario Austral de Valdivia" of 23 August 1978 (see Salazar and Pinto 1999: 165).

communities suffered abuse, arrest, torture and murder on suspicion of being Allende supporters (ibid.: 2). As pointed out by Sergio Caniuqueo, however, many Mapuche also sought alliances with the right, and declared unconditional support for the military regime (Caniuqueo 2006; Crow 2013: 157). To some degree the right also celebrated Mapuche identity, for instance through teaching programmes for rural Mapuche and through articles about Mapuche culture and history (Crow 2013: 174).

As part of Pinochet's neo-liberal economic politics, a highly capital-intensive, commercial type of farming developed in the rural areas based on pine plantations subsidized by the state.[13] This new type of agriculture produced economic growth, but also led to an intensification of rural poverty among the Mapuche (Luna 2007: 103). As a consequence of the politics of the military regime, the majority of the Mapuche population moved to the cities,[14] and employment on farms that had used wage labour was largely replaced by work in construction and service.

MODERN CHILE: ENTERING DEMOCRACY

In 1989 democracy was reintroduced to Chile after an election in which the majority of the Chilean population voted against the military regime, to the latter's surprise. The same year, authors Joaquín Lavín and Luis Larraín claimed that Chile had become "a more efficient society, more humane, better informed, more cultured" (cited in Collier and Sater 2004: 375). They pointed to the reality of modern Chile, where huge shopping malls, supermarkets and consumer goods presented material signs that modernization had arrived. American-style malls, big shopping centres with a "feel good" atmosphere, emphasized the pleasures of consuming in a clean, orderly and secure atmosphere guaranteed by the security guard in front of each shop, which was conducive to a feeling of complete "safety" in all parts of the multifunctional space. They contain an abundance of leisure options: cinemas, restaurants, playgrounds or play equipment for children and a large variety of shops. Families use them for weekend trips: the children play in the play areas and buy ice-creams, and a meal can be

[13] According to a study by CORA (Corporacion de Reforma Agraria), in 1969 it was estimated that a Mapuche family would be able to live a "dignified" life with 50 hectares of land; at the end of the century, the average size of a plot of land for a Mapuche family was 3 hectares.

[14] According to PNUD (Programa de las Naciones Unidas para el Desarollo), 79.2% of the Mapuche live in urban areas (PNUD 2000: 63).

had for a reasonable price in the restaurants. This seems like a consumer's paradise, offering the type of recreational activity which forms a crucial part of everyday life for many middle-class Chileans. Here it is possible to fulfil the dream of the modern citizen of equipping the house with all that is necessary for a contemporary, well-functioning family: telephone, television (one for each room), refrigerator, cooker, microwave oven, mobile telephone, washing machine, DVD, video, music centre, computer, clothes, shoes and cosmetics (Moulian 1997: 113). After the transition to democracy in 1990, subsequent democratic governments[15] chose not to alter the basic free-market organization of Chile's economy, so as not to tamper with this popular model of consumption.

Of interest to this study, however, are the effects that the neo-liberal model of the free market has had on Chilean society in relation to cultural identity and class relations. Among the analyses of the socio-political situation in the country, it is not very difficult to find voices of critique. In his book *Chile Actual: Anatomía de un mito* (Contemporary Chile: Anatomy of a Myth, 1997), sociologist Tomás Moulian draws a pessimistic picture of the Chilean nation-state and analyses the so-called *matriz*[16] (matrix, origins) of the Chilean way of living. He describes the Chilean lifestyle as characterized by a postmodern lack of ideologies and values, the outcome of a neo-liberal model where all forms of collective action were suspended and replaced with capitalist, free-market politics. The aim was to provide "freedom" for the consumer without the restrictions that arise from having an active labour union movement. This was replaced by the "right of the consumer" to buy and consume whatever he or she wants. Consequently, "consumption" became the new ideology of the Chileans, which, according to Moulian, "surpasses income and therefore requires a contract of debt" (Moulian 1997: 104). As the income of an average Chilean is insufficient to cover consumption demands, a collective

---

[15] That is, the governments of Patricio Aylwin (1990–1994), Eduardo Frei Ruiz-Tagle (1994–2000), Ricardo Lagos (2000–2006), Michelle Bachelet (2006–2010) and Sebastian Piñera (2010–2014).

[16] The metaphor of the *matriz* expresses the idea of a lineage and the assumption that to be a product of specific semen and womb is to have the effects of these inscribed into the body, the character, the history. Or, in other words, the type of container defines the content. In this way, body and society are defined as formed by the same space, which can be more or less rigid or flexible. In the case of Chile this is referred to as the materialization of the strategies of the military and neo-liberal intellectuals as well as national and trans-national managers (Moulian 1997: 17).

solution has become acceptable: plastic money or credit cards, which is why Moulian refers to the Chilean as "El ciudadano credit-card" (the credit-card citizen; Moulian 1997: 102). Department stores such as Alamacenes Paris and Falabella not only offer credit cards, they have also opened banks (Han 2012: 32). Credit cards have become the solution to the uneven distribution of wealth. For the lower classes, the possibility of buying on credit facilitates acquisition of the goods that have become the emblems of a satisfactory modern life. The credit card has become both a resource and a sign of identity, connecting the individual to the notion of "leisure". One year of work at the minimum wage of 100,000 pesos is the prerequisite for entering this "paradise of consumption". Being accepted as a credit card holder is tantamount to being considered a worthy citizen and worker; it is the ticket to modernity for those who cannot pay in cash. It is, consequently, closely tied to the notion of materiality, the objects through which the subject constructs the self. The plastic card has a double function, both as the medium through which the performance of identity can be displayed—enjoying the pleasures of life—and as a medium to discipline workers, because it is a means of controlling the consumer, a way of regulating the body of the worker. They seem to have been given the possibility of living the comfortable modern life. Only one problem remains: the money used has to be paid back. What at first looks like the door to freedom and pleasure becomes a trap, the "purgatory of indebtedness" (Moulian 1997: 89).

Backed by hard data from his own and others' research, Moulian argues that credit cards entice their users into becoming part of the "consumers' paradise", but also serve to cover up serious social inequalities in democratic Chile (1997: 102–104). According to him, Chile presents an example of increasingly unequal income distribution compared with the time before the military regime. Likewise, other authors argue that the economic model of the military regime has served to reduce poverty, but increased inequalities in the distribution of wealth (Collier and Sater 2004; Loveman 2001). Indeed, the flip side of economic growth is intensification of urban and rural poverty. The poorest two-fifths of the population and sections of the middle class have to cope with static and even declining living standards. What is even more interesting, however, is that in the democratic governments following Pinochet's regime, social inequalities have not decreased. In 1994 a person with an average high annual income ($441,749) earned about 40 times more than the average low income ($11,131). According to Borzutsky and Oppenheim, the poorest 10% of the population receives 1.3% of the wealth, in contrast to the richest 10% of the population, who receive 41% (2006: xix–xx). In 2006 the national census showed that low-income populations with an income between $110 and $300 per month spend 36% of their monthly income on consumer debt (MIDEPLAN 2006 in Han 2012: 32). Moreover, as described in Chap. 3, access to public services and health care is characterized by insufficient resources, poor infrastructure and a lack of medical equipment and medicine (Borzutsky and Oppenheim 2006: 150–151; Han 2012). As also noted by Richards (2013), although neo-liberal reforms have generally upheld political and civil rights, social rights to public services such as health care and education have largely been downsized. In other words, an important aspect of neo-liberalism has been the delegation of what were previously state responsibilities to non-governmental and community organizations. In consequence, the role of citizens, indigenous and non-indigenous, has been reduced to voting, consuming and participating in community projects (Richards 2013: 10).

THE MAPUCHE IN POST-DICTATORSHIP CHILE

According to Richards, there is never complete consensus in collective memory (Richards 2013: 33). Her argument accords with the findings of this study that different groups in Chile adhere to competing narratives about the past, and also possess varying visions of the future. The neo-liberal model of the military regime had serious political and economic consequences. First and foremost, as already indicated, there was no recognition of the existence of Chile's indigenous minorities; the Mapuche were especially alarmed by the effects of the expansion of private timber companies into indigenous communities. In many areas indigenous lands became extremely eroded and water resources scarce due to the encroachment of numerous pinewood plantations, as pines absorb huge amounts of water which leads to the impoverishment of an area's biodiversity (Kristensen 1999, 2000).

On the other hand, the reintroduction of democracy became a starting point for national self-reflection and a search for roots. Civil society, which had been frozen in Pinochet's iron grip, regained the possibility to express itself and to act, and Pinochet's idea of the homogenous white population was questioned. During the election campaign that ousted Pinochet, the candidate of the Christian Democratic Party, Patricio Aylwin, met the most important representatives of Chile's indigenous people in the city of Nuevo Imperial. A contract was signed with a commitment to work for a fairer policy for indigenous people in the transition to democracy (Bengoa 1999: 184). Changes were slow to materialize, however, as right-wing elements still had the majority in parliament, and in 1992 the 500th anniversary of Columbus's discovery of the Americas was marked by a major demonstration.

During the government of Eduardo Frei (1994–2000), the Indigenous Law 19.253 of 1993 represented a new era, as it guaranteed that "territory defined as indigenous will enjoy protection from the act and cannot be disposed of, confiscated, encumbered nor acquired through prescription except between communities or indigenous individuals of the same ethnic group" (Article 13). According to the law, indigenous people who can prove direct kinship with persons who were granted the right to a territory (via the so-called Titulo de Merced, discussed earlier) between 1884 and 1927 can rightfully claim to be the owners of the land. The governmental institution of indigenous people, CONADI (la Corporacíon Nacional de Desarollo Indígena/the State Agency for Indigenous People), was granted funds and the authorization to take over the purchase of the 150,000 hectares of land subsequently transferred to the Mapuche. However, the funds allocated were only sufficient to buy a fraction of what the Mapuche had lost under Pinochet's dictatorship to private land owners and timber companies (Aylwin 2000: 5). Furthermore, Frei's government gave the green light to the construction of six hydroelectric dams on indigenous land, as well as offering subsidies to multinational companies. At the end of Frei's government the multinational companies owned 1.5 million hectares of land, while the Mapuche owned 500,000 hectares.[17]

From 1994 to 2005, CONADI bought a total of 406,666 hectares of land worth a total of $142 million, land which was transferred to indigenous peoples. Of this, 200,000 hectares of land went to the Mapuche (Aylwin 2007). Another significant improvement was the introduction of scholarships for indigenous peoples, and from 2000 to 2005 a total of 152,317 fellowships were awarded. Nevertheless, these initiatives did not solve the social and political problems. While poverty among the Chilean population, according to official figures from 2001, was 22.7%, among the indigenous inhabitants it was 35.6% (World Bank 2001, cited in Stavenhagen 2003). An indigenous family received 50% of what was classed as the normal income for a Chilean family and only 3% of the rural population had completed long-term education (ibid.).

[17] "El Mercurio", 15 January 1999.

THE MAPUCHE MOVEMENT AND THE ALTERNATIVE
TO MODERNITY

Since the 1990s, a Mapuche social movement has developed that challenges the official version of history and the ideological order and has as its objective the recovery of the territories originally granted to the Mapuche under the Titulo de Merced that have fallen into the hands of timber companies and private farmers. Other sources of conflict have been the building of hydroelectric dams, airports, highways, corporate fisheries and garbage dumps (Richards 2013: 76). In 1997 various Mapuche organizations initiated a process that became known as "the territorial recuperation", whose goal it was to recover 400,000 hectares of land. From that year onwards, the terms "conflict" and "violence" began to colour the relationship between the Chilean government, private companies and the Mapuche. In December 1997 in the province of Lumaco, three trucks belonging to the Aurauco timber company were set on fire. Eleven people, all Mapuche, were imprisoned under the Chilean anti-terror law dating from Pinochet's epoch, which suspends normal judicial practice.[18] In spite of a clear lack of evidence, the prisoners were detained for months. They began a hunger strike that gained them rising support outside the prison walls. The "conflict", as it was labelled by the Chilean press and the government, was regarded by a number of academics, as well as the Mapuche themselves, as a symbol of the social injustice to which the Mapuche were exposed.

In February 1998, leading figures from the Mapuche movement appeared in the media, including Aucán Huilcamán, spokesperson for the organization "El Consejo de Todas las Tierras", and Víctor Ancalaf, spokesperson for the organization "La Coordinadora". They designated 1998 a year of protest and the start of the Mapuche struggle, both for recognition as a people and for the recovery of 400,000 hectares of land. In response, the timber companies intensified the burning of trees on native land, provoking a strong reaction. Throughout Southern Chile, the Mapuche, motivated by the right to land granted by the Titulo de Merced, occupied large numbers of *fundos*, or haciendas, owned by the timber companies in the region. In addition to territory being occupied, highways were blocked, bridges cut and machines burned. These actions gave rise to violent clashes between employees from the timber companies, private farmers and the Mapuche. Scenes from the conflict mirrored those of a civil war, with the

---

[18] "El Diario Austral", 10 December 1997.

Mapuche (including women, children and elderly people) armed with stones and wooden clubs facing a heavily armed police force equipped with tanks, police dogs and tear gas, sent in to protect the timber companies' property. Several areas were declared a state of emergency.

If we look at events from 1997 onwards, the conclusion can be drawn that all exhibit violence as a pivotal point. From the viewpoint of the Chilean government, the Mapuche movement was primarily considered a protest against marginalization and poverty in rural areas. At the same time, however, the movement was seen as a threat to public security and described as both "violent" and an example of modern terrorism. It was widely rumoured that in order to be able to sign a free trade agreement with the USA, getting the Mapuche movement under control was set as a precondition (Richards 2013: 108). Consequently, a very hard line was taken, one that was framed by anti-terrorism laws.

For the timber companies, whose large-scale export of timber contributes substantially to Chile's general economy, economic growth and profit margins are among the prime considerations. Yet their activities were threatened due to what was referred to as systematic activities of terrorism and vandalism against employees and their private property. On these grounds the forestry companies, supported by right-wing politicians, urged the Chilean government to take action against the "Mapuche terrorists" in order to secure the economy and avoid an abyss of horror like the Mexican Chiapas or the guerrilla wars in Columbia.

The Chilean press has largely supported the timber companies' version of events by stressing the violent activities of the so-called Mapuche terrorists. From the beginning of the conflict, phrases such as "spiralling violence", "rural terrorism", "brutal assault" and "racial conflict" became part of the newspapers' vocabulary. In addition, various newspapers propagated the idea of a guerrilla war organized by radical Marxists with foreign support and funding.[19] They also depicted a possible future with the country divided into two nations. In order to prevent a civil war, they called on the Chilean government to take measures against "the terrorists" by, for example, applying the anti-terrorism law. According to an opinion poll published in "La Tercera", however, this view did not gain much support in the Chilean capital of Santiago. More than 80% of the respondents agreed that the territories legitimately belonged to the

[19] "El Sur", 2 February 2000.

Mapuche, and 68% considered the means used by the Mapuche movement to obtain its goals legitimate.[20]
Finally, according to the Mapuche movement, the violence was a
response to an oppressive state apparatus, the cruelties perpetrated under
the dictatorship of Pinochet and those committed by Spaniards and
Chileans against the Mapuche since colonization, as well as the injustice
caused by capitalism and neo-liberalism. The victims of the political economy have been the Mapuche who, according to statistics, are among the
most marginalized groups in Chile, with low levels of income and high
levels of infant mortality, malnutrition, unemployment and illiteracy
(Kristensen 2000: 143).

Since 1997, confrontations between private landowners, the Mapuche
and the military have continued and, to this day, Chilean prisons are filled
with Mapuche with sentences of up to 20 years. During police raids people
have been subjected to verbal abuse, and cases of torture have been
reported. Limbs have been broken, and pregnant women have lost unborn
babies due to violence (Richards 2013: 126). To protest against the use of
anti-terrorist laws, Mapuche prisoners have undertaken several hunger
strikes. Patricia Troncoso, who was sentenced to 10 years for arson in association with fires on a pine plantation owned by Mininco, fasted for
112 days in January 2008, before finally being granted weekend leaves and
access to the rural outdoors (Richards 2013: 106). In comparison, there
has been no form of judicial settlement in connection with the killing of
Mapuche in clashes between police and demonstrations, such as the murder of 17-year-old Alex Lemun by police officers during a demonstration.
In response to these incidents, in 2003 the UN Special Rapporteur on the
rights of indigenous peoples, Rudolf Stavenhagen, strongly criticized the
use of the anti-terrorist law, noting in a report that "activities in the form
of protests and social demands should not be criminalized or punished"
(Stavenhagen 2003: 69–70). Human Rights Watch (2004), El
Observatorio de Derechos de los Pueblos Indigenas (2004) and the UN
Human Rights Committee also published highly critical reports. However,
so far this has not led to any significant changes in the political line taken
against the Mapuche movement.

The "Mapuche conflict" has revealed deep tensions in contemporary
Chile. As phrased by Patricia Richards, "Politically persecuted, economically exploited, racially oppressed, the Mapuche are now paying the envi-

[20] "La Tercera", 18 April 1999.

ronmental consequences of national development" (Richards 2013: 2). In this context, Mapuche identity politics and demands for land represent resistance, opposition and an alternative to the political neo-liberal project. The Mapuche are forcing themselves onto the social stage as subjects and demanding to be recognized as a distinct people (Richards 2010: 85). Meanwhile, machis are coming to be regarded as "symbols of tradition", as they possess the spiritual knowledge connected to the territory (Bacigalupo 2007); they have, therefore, been key figures in protests and demonstrations. Chilean governments view the politicization of machis as a threat to the state (Bacigalupo 2016: 189); for this reason, several machis have been persecuted.

It is interesting to note that the process of the recovery of territory, initially a protest against the marginalization and impoverishment of the Mapuche, has increasingly become a political project that counters the neo-liberal projects of the state (de la Cadena 2010). The Mapuche activists regard the process as resistance and decolonization, whose aims are to restore historical memory and political consciousness and gain auto-determination as a people (Boccara 2002; Pairican 2012, 2015). The political protests have been accompanied by critical analysis of colonial history and violence from a Mapuche perspective (Caniuqueo 2006), in order to make visible Mapuche ethnic difference in the Chilean collective imagery; the result of this, they claim, should be their political recognition as a people rather than the application of development-oriented solutions. Mapuche intellectuals have supported activism as a defence against the devalorization of tradition and identity, and the intent to homogenize the culture in the context of globalization, capitalism and neo-liberalism (Pairican 2015: 312–313).

Conclusion: Tensions and Forgetting in the New Chile

In 1992, a piece of ice from the Chilean Antarctica was transported to Seville to appear in the event "la Feria Universal Expo Sevilla 92". The iceberg was presented as a symbol of the new Chile, totally negating the country's indigenous roots and its violent past. Chile was presented as a white country, without memory and origins, cleansed by its prolonged stay in the sea. In the iceberg all traces of the blood of those who were lost forever had been crystallized into a deep blue; their agonies had become the white veins of the ice, without even a trace of the shadow of Pinochet. The iceberg was a symbol of a born-again Chile (Moulian 1997: 31–37). In Chile the olvidos have been intertwined in a political system that to marginalized and vulnerable people is perceived as a political "system of torture", where everyday challenges and bodily pains are normalized and taken as part and parcel of the physical experience of living (as also argued by Clara Han 2012: 19, 27). However, as is argued in this present work, the olvido—the forgetting in the new Chile of the past—is in no way absolute. The olvidos appear as examples of the "uncanny", as theorized by Freud: things which ought to have remained hidden but have come to light. That is, the apparently forgotten and repressed is articulated and negotiated in an alternative framework for remembering—in this case, in medical practice and illness symptoms. In the following chapters I explore how indigenous medical practice might also represent a possible solution for "otherness". What might appear as reminiscent of a past that is long gone makes its presence felt in the constant negotiation and reproduction of the missing past, the suppressed identities, and cultural and political activities. It is the links between stories of medical practice and socio-political processes which this work seeks to examine: the embodiment of the historical structure of the nation-state that relies on certain processes of memory and forgetting.

REFERENCES

Anderson, Benedict. 1983. *Imagined Communities*. London: Verso.
Arana, Diego Barros. 1884. *Historia de Chile*. Santiago de Chile: Ediciones Rafel Jover.
Arana, Diego Barros. 1934. *Origines de Chile: Los Fundamentos de la Nacionalidad*. Santiago de Chile: Editorial Nascimiento.
Aylwin, José. 2000. Los Conflictos en el Territorio Mapuche: Antecedentes y Perspectivas. *Revista Perspectivas* 3(2).
Aylwin, José. 2007. La política del "nuevo trato": Antecedentes, alcances y limitaciones. *El gobierno de Lagos, los pueblos indígenas y el "nuevo trato"*. Santiago: *LOM Ediciones*.
Bacigalupo, Ana Mariella. 2007. *Thunder Shaman. Making History with Mapuche Spirits in Chile and Patagonia*. Texas: University of Texas Press.
Bacigalupo, Ana Mariella. 2016. *Shamans of the Foye Tree. Gender, Power, and Healing among Chilean Mapuche*. Texas: University of Texas Press.
Bengoa, José. 1985. *Historia del Pueblo Mapuche*. Santiago de Chile: Ediciones Sur Coleccion.

Bengoa, José. 1999. *Historia de un Conflicto: El Estado y los Mapuches en el Siglo XX*. Planeta SA.

Boccara, Guillaume. 2002. The Mapuche People in Post-Dictatorship Chile. *Ètudes Rurales*. No. 163/164. Terre Territoire Appartenances: 283–303.

Boccara, G. & Seguel-Boccara, I. 1999. Políticas indígenas en Chile (Siglos XIX y XX). De la asimilación al pluralismo (El caso mapuche). *Revista de Indias* 59(217): 741–774.

Borzutsky, Silvia. 2006. Cooperation or Confrontation between State and the Market: Social Security and Health Policies. In: Silvia Borzutsky & Lois Hecht Oppenheim (eds.), *After Pinochet: The Chilean Road to Democracy and the Market*. Gainesville: University Press of Florida, pp. 142–166.

Borzutsky, Silvia & Lois Hecht Oppenheim. 2006. Introduction. In: Silvia Borzutsky & Lois Hecht Oppenheim (eds.), *After Pinochet: The Chilean Road to Democracy and the Market*. Gainesville: University Press of Florida, pp. xiiv–xxv.

Canclini, Nestór García. 1989. *Culturas Híbridas: Estrategias para Entrar y Salir de la Modernidad*. Santiago de Chile: Editorial Grijalbo.

Caniuqueo, Sergio. 2006. Siglo XX en Gulumapu: De la fragmentación del Wallmapu a la unidad nacional Mapuche. 1880 a 1978. In: Pablo Marimán, Sergio Caniuqueo, José Millalén, Rodrigo level. Eschucha Winka. Cuatro ensayos de Historia Nacional Mapuche y un epílogo sobre el futuro. Satiago, Lom Ediciones, pp. 129–218.

Citarella, Luca, et al. 1995. *Medicinas y Cultura en la Araucanía*. Santiago de Chile: Editorial Sudamericana.

Collier, Simon. 1996. *A History of Chile 1808–1994*. Cambridge: Cambridge University Press.

Collier, Simon & William F. Sater. 2004. *A History of Chile, 1808–2002*. Cambridge: Cambridge University Press.

Crow, Joanna. 2013. *The Mapuche in modern Chile: A cultural history*. University Press of Florida.

De la Cadena, M. 2010. Indigenous cosmopolitics in the Andes: Conceptual reflections beyond "politics". *Cultural Anthropology* 25(2): 334–370.

de Moesbach, E.W. & P. Coña. 2000 [1930]. *Vida y costumbres de los indígenas araucanos en la segunda mitad del siglo XIX*. Impr. Cervantes.

Ercilla, Alonso de. 1982. *Araucania*. Santiago de Chile: Editorial Andres Bello.

Foerster, Rolf. 1993. *Introducción a la Religiosidad Mapuche*. Santiago de Chile: Editorial Universitaria.

Foerster, Rolf. 1996. *Jesuitas y Mapuches 1593–1767*. Santiago: Editorial Universitaria.

Foerster, Rolf & Sonia Montecino. 1988. *Organizaciones, Líderes y Contiendas Mapuche* (1900–1979). Santiago de Chile: CEM.

Giminiani, Piergiorgio Di. 2012. *Tierras ancestrales, disputas contemporáneas. Perteninencia y demandas territoriales en la sociedad mapuche rural*. Santiago: Ediciones Universidad Católica de Chile.

Gonzales Galves, Marcelo Ignacio. 2012. Personal Truths, Shared Equivocations. Otherness, Uniqueness, and Social Life among the Mapuche of Southern Chile. PhD in Social Anthropology. The University of Edinburgh.

Guevara, Tomas. 1913. Las Ultimas Familas y Costumbres Araucanas. Santiago: Imprente, Litografía I Encuadernacion "Barcelona".

Han, Clara. 2004. The Work of Indebtedness: The Traumatic Present of Late Capitalist Chile. *Culture, Medicine and Psychiatry* 28(2): 169–187.

Han, Clara. 2012. *Life in Debt. Times of Care and Violence in Neoliberal Chile*. London: University of California Press.

Jones, Kristine. 1999. The Southern Margin (1673–1882). In: Frank Salomon & Stuart Schwartz (eds.), *The Cambridge History of Native People of the Americas*. Volume 3, South America part 2. New York. Cambridge University Press, pp. 140–181.

Kristensen, Dorthe Brogård. 1999. Chile. In: *The Indigenous World 1998–1999*. København: Iwgia, pp. 121–124.

Kristensen, Dorthe Brogård. 2000. Chile. In: *The Indigenous World 1999–2000*. København: Iwgia, pp. 142–148.

Lincoqueo, José Huenuman. 2002. Genocidio, Cabello de Troya de Mefistífeles (El Demonios). Análisis Jurídico acerca de los Parlamentos. In: Carlos Contreras Painemal (ed.), *Actas del Primer Congreso Internacional de Historia Mapuche*. UKE Mapufórlaget, pp. 70–76.

Loveman, Brian. 2001. *Chile: The Legacy of Hispanic Capitalism*. New York and Oxford: Oxford University Press.

Luna, L. 2007. *Un mundo entre dos mundos: las relaciones entre el pueblo mapuche y el estado chileno desde la perspectiva del desarrollo y de los cambios sociocultura-les*. Sede Villarrica: Pontificia Universidad Católica de Chile.

Mallon, F.E. 2005. *Courage tastes of blood: The Mapuche community of Nicolás Ailío and the Chilean state, 1906–2001*. Duke University Press.

Marimán, Pablo. 2006. Los mapuche antes de la conquista militar chileno-argentina. In: Pablo Marimán, Sergio Caniuqueo, José Millalén, Rodrigo level. Eschucha Winka. Cuatro ensayos de Historia Nacional Mapuche y un epílogo sobre el futuro. Satiago: Lom Ediciones, pp. 53–128.

Mariqueo, Reynaldo. 1989. *The Etno-Development of the Mapuche People*. IWGIA document no. 63. IWGIA: Copenhagen.

Moulian, Tomás. 1997. *Anatomía de un Mito*. Arcis Universidad: LOM Ediciones, Serie Punto de Fga. Coleccion sin Norte.

Nájera, Alfonso Gonzáles de. 1971. *Desengaño y reparo de la guerra del reino de Chile*. Santiago de Chile: Editorial Andres Bello.

Ovalle, Alonso de. 2003 (1646). *Historia relacion del reino de Chile*. Santiago de Chile: Pehuén. Biblioteca del Bicentenario.

Pairican, Fernando Padilla. 2012. Sembrando ideología: el Aukiñ Wallmapu Ngulam in the transition of Aylwin (1990–1994). *Sudhistoria* 4: 12–42.

Pairican, Fernando Padilla. 2015. El retorno de un viejo actor político: el guerrero. Perspectivas para comprender la violencia política en el movimiento mapuche (1990–2010). In *Violencia coloniales en Wallmapu*. Centro de Estudios y Investigaciones Mapuche, pp. 301–324.

Paley, Julia. 2001. *Marketing Democracy: Power and Social Movements in Post-dictatorship Chile*. London: University of California Press.

Pinto, Jorge. 2000. *De la inclusión a la exclusión. La formación del estado, la nación y el pueblo mapuche*. Santiago: Universidad de Santiago.

PNUD. 2000. *Desarrollo humano en Chile 2000: Mas sociedad para gobernar el futuro*.

Rahier, Jean Muteba. 2003. Introduction: *Mestizaje, Mulataje, Mestiçagem* in Latin American Ideologies of National Identities. *Journal of Latin American Anthropology* 8(1): 40–51.

Richards, P. 2010. Of Indians and terrorists: how the state and local elites construct the Mapuche in neoliberal multicultural Chile. *Journal of Latin American Studies* 42(1): 59–90.

Richards, P. 2013. *Race and the Chilean miracle: Neoliberalism, democracy, and indigenous rights*. University of Pittsburgh Press.

Rosales, Diego. 1989 (1674). *Historia general del reino de Chile*. Valparaiso: Imprenta de El Mercurio.

Salazar, Gabriel & Julio Pinto. 1999. *Historia contemporánea de Chile II: Actores, identidad y movimiento*. Santiago: LOM Ediciones.

Schamis, Hector E. 2002. *Reforming the State: The Politics of Privatization in Latin America and Europe*. Ann Arbor: The University of Michigan Press.

Stavenhagen, Rodolfo. 2003. Informe del Relator Especial sobre la situación de los derechos humanos y las libertades fundamentales de los indígenas, presentado de conformidad con la resolución 2003/56 de la Comisión.

Valdivia, Luis. 1621. Sermon en lengva de Chile, de los mysterios de nvestra santa fe catholica, para dedicarla a los indios infieles del reyno de Chile, dividido en nveve partes pequeñas, acomodadas a ſu capacidad.

CHAPTER 3

Complex Illnesses and Complementary Cures

The medical context in Southern Chile is characterized by a range of practices that include biomedicine, Mapuche medicine, Christian evangelical healers, Bach medicine, acupuncture and spiritualist healing (as noted in Chap. 1). The historical background of this situation is based on the existence of medical pluralism in the area as well as the dynamics of local power relations: between the state and public medical practices on the one hand, and indigenous medical practices on the other. This pluralism is also characterized by the parallel use of, and interchange between, medical traditions, in this case between indigenous medicine and the medical traditions of the missionaries. This chapter takes its point of departure from an analysis of the historical background of the medical context, in which it is shown how the missionaries and Mapuche co-existed and adopted some of each other's practices in the field of illness treatment. This came to an end in the 1920s when public health was introduced and officially became the only legal medical alternative, although citizens who identified both as Mapuche and Chileans continued to combine different types of healing. The initial analysis of the context of medical pluralism serves as a backdrop for the presentation of scenes from contemporary Chile that follow, including discussion of the case of a mestizo, Sonia, who used both biomedicine and Mapuche medicine to treat her depression. This links to the notion of personhood in the south of Chile, where illness narratives, medical dialogues and social relationships are means through which people create themselves (Course 2011).

© The Author(s) 2019   63
D. B. Kristensen, *Patients, Doctors and Healers*,
https://doi.org/10.1007/978-3-319-97031-8_3

Early documents produced by the missionaries mention a number of indigenous specialists—*ngutanfe*, who dealt with wounds and bone fractures, and *kupofe kupon* or surgeons—but the ritual and medical experts of the Mapuche, the machis, were described as more important figures who dealt with overall health (Latcham 1928).[1] Machis, who were initiated through dreams and trance states, combined the use of herbal remedies and healing rituals with diagnosis, surgery and bone-setting; they also carried out autopsies and divination (Bacigalupo 2007: 117). Traditionally machis played only a minor role in collective rituals such as *nguillatun*, a fertility ritual that was and still is the largest and most important event in Mapuche communities (Foerster 1993: 116; Latcham 1924: 677; Course 2011: 138). It was once headed by the *lonko* (chief) of the community, but increasingly machis have taken over this role. In colonial times machis also played an important role in war time. Before a battle with the colonizers, the machis performed a ritual wherein they asked the ancestor spirit for protection and advice and blew tobacco towards the land of their enemies as a curse. They also divined the location of the Spanish soldiers and the outcomes of confrontations by performing magic in bowls of water (Rosales 1989: 135; Bacigalupo 2007: 118) According to Latcham, the Mapuche called upon pillan, the spirits of warriors that have turned into volcanoes and that can cross the sea and assist in war; the common belief is that thunder is produced by pillan battles above the sky (Latcham 1928: 194; Rosales 1989 [1674]: 162–163). There are both good pillan, the souls of the Mapuche that reside in volcanoes, and evil, those of the Spanish colonizers. In a similar way, the Spaniards believed that Christian forces were important actors in wartime, for example that the Virgin Mary blinded the Mapuche warriors with light and dust (Ercilla y Zúñiga 1933 in Bacigalupo 2007: 117).

Despite the constant warfare between Mapuche and Spaniards, their medical practices mutually developed through the interaction. In the early colonial period, Spanish medicine did not have a scientific base, but was largely founded on religious practices. Thus, many similarities could be found between indigenous medicine and the medicine of the European settlers, and indigenous herbal remedies were incorporated into the pharmacy of the missionaries. Medical education was initiated in Chile with the foundation of the University of San Felipe and taught by Spanish missionaries in the first period of colonization, which was characterized by the presence of

---

[1] Interview with Juan Ñanculef, see Latcham (1924: 435).

the Jesuits (Cruz-Coke 1992). Indeed, the Jesuit missionaries developed relationships with the native population by virtue of the interchange of information and practices connected with healing (Foerster 1996: 260). Consequently, in their attempts to evangelize or convert the indigenous population, the Jesuits adopted many of its practices (Pinto 1988; Foerster 1996). For instance, they used exorcizing techniques similar to the machis and in some cases holy water to heal the sick (Bacigalupo 2007: 121). Yet, although some practices were similar, there were also crucial differences, for instance although the Jesuits perceived relics and rosarios to be saintly, they regarded machi drums as instruments of witchcraft (Bacigalupo 2007: 129).

Conversely, the indigenous population adopted Spanish and Christian practices, such as baptism and the use of the cross, in a syncretism between Christianity and Mapuche religion (Citarella et al. 1995: 430; Foerster 1993: 263). A missionary describes how the indigenous population even sought the medical assistance of a priest when one of their own medical practitioners (their machi) was ill; this priest performed a ritual of exorcism through an invocation in the name of Jesus and by using a relic (from the picture of Saint Ignacio; Pinto 1988: 56–58, cited in Citarella et al. 1995: 430). This vignette illustrates the historical process of syncretism between Mapuche and Spanish practices, which has continuity in many current medical and religious practices, such as the use of the Christian cross and holy water in the fertility ritual *nguillatun*, and the use of the cross and invocation of Christian saints in shamanistic healing rituals (discussed in more detail in Chap. 7).

The Catholic Church and the Jesuits constituted the most powerful order of all, owning over 50 estates, the only pharmacies and the hospital. In 1767 the Spanish Empire decided to expel the Jesuits from its colonies and 400 Jesuits were deported from Chile, in one of the most dramatic events of the period. This put an end to the close relationship between the Jesuits and the native population (Collier and Sater 2004: 22) and also led to the deterioration of medical development, as the Jesuits represented the cultural elite of the country and had the best professionals and libraries (Cruz-Coke 1992). The marked shortage of medical doctors which resulted was a severe handicap in the fight against smallpox and other epidemics. Afterwards, missionary work in the Spanish Empire was handed over to the Franciscans, who were convinced that the best way to evangelize the natives was to "erase" indigenous belief completely, a project which derived from their idea of the effectiveness of the tabula rasa or blank slate (Foerster 1993: 34). As part of this strategy they projected their very negative perceptions of the indigenous religion, which they considered "demonic". These developments did not, however, prevent the continuation of syncretism; the adoption of Christian elements into the Mapuche religion and of Mapuche religious and medical practices among the Spaniards was unabated (Foerster 1993: 47). After the integration of the indigenous population in the south between 1881 and 1884, missionaries continued their work in the area and the indigenous population responded to the presence of the missionaries by further integrating Christian elements into their practices.[2]

In the first decades after the national integration of the Mapuche, very few medical doctors ventured into the area—due to both interethnic strife and very low remuneration (Citarella et al. 1995: 444)—and, in their absence, the colonizers also made use of Mapuche healing practices (Dufey in Caniuqueo 2006: 153). With the introduction of the public health system in Chile from the 1920s, however, medicine in Chile became part of a public discourse wherein only one medicine, biomedicine, was officially recognized.

PUBLIC HEALTH IN CHILE: AN INTRODUCTION

The literature on the development of public health in Chile, especially with regard to the period of the military regime, is relatively sparse and mostly restricted to official documents and a few historical analyses by local Chilean scholars (Citarella et al. 1995; Giaconi 1994; Miranda 1994) and foreign historians (Borzutsky 2006). Public health in Chile originated in an attempt by the Spanish Crown to control the activities of health practitioners, whereby it was stated that only persons with a degree from an officially recognized university were allowed to work as doctors. This control continues to constitute the legal framework for practising medicine in Chile, which is established in the so-called Codigo Sanitaria (Sanitary Code).[3] Despite the regulations, first by the Spanish Crown and thereafter by the Chilean state, biomedicine was not very developed and for that reason did not play a major role in the medical practices of the population in the south of Chile until the 1920s. Therefore the colonos

---

[2] An example of this is the practice of the so-called *nguillatún-misa*, a combination of a Christian mass and the Mapuche ritual of fertility, *nguillatun*, where a sheep was sacrificed as the "symbol of God" while a bishop (in this case, Monseñor Guido de Ramberg) blessed the food and drink (described in Forster and Montecino 1996: 63).

[3] Law Decree no. 725, published 31 January 1968.

continued to make use of Mapuche medicine (Caniuqueo 2006: 155). From 1920 to 1940 state programmes and health insurance to cover the needs of the population (i.e. the workers) were introduced (for instance, the Ley de Seguridad Social; Citarella et al. 1995: 438–439). In 1952 the Servicio Nacional de Salud (National Health Service) and, in 1968, the Servicio Medico Nacional de Empleados (National Health Service for Workers) were created as governmental instruments to address—free of charge—the health problems of the majority of the population. By 1973, about 75% of the population was covered by the social security system (Borzutsky 2006: 143).

During the military regime, however, the health system underwent major changes, mainly consisting of a drastic reduction of the role of the state, and in 1979–1980 reforms instigating the privatization of social security were introduced. In addition, the National Health Service was decentralized, leaving its administration to the local municipalities (Citarella et al. 1995: 489–490; Collier and Sater 2004: 374; Miranda 1994: 58–59; Giaconi 1994: 257–273). The health system was divided into a public health system—the Sistema Nacional de Servicios de Salud, covered by a public system of health insurance FONASA (Fondo Nacional de Salud)—and a private health system, mainly supported by private health insurance. In 1981 the private insurance system known as ISAPRES (Instituciones de Salud Previsional)[4] was introduced and in 1985 free maternity and emergency health services were abolished (*Organización Panamericana de la Salud* 2002: 78). The stated goal of the creation of this mixed system was to give the user the freedom to choose between public and private health services. In reality it became a system that was based on the ability of the user to purchase effective health insurance; in other words, quality and accessibility depended on income, with the best services provided in the private sector. The state system was thus assigned responsibility for the lower social strata.

With the introduction of democracy, the mixed health system inherited from the military regime was in large part maintained, with a few changes, such as the introduction of national regulation and control over private health insurance. Today, public health insurance has become the most widespread (and cheapest) option, used by 62% of the Chilean population

---

[4] ISAPRES are "private entities that offer a series of medical insurance and workman's compensation packages in return for a basic 7% payroll contribution plus an additional premium of 2–3% depending on the size of the package" (Borzutsky 2006: 150).

(a figure which corresponds with the lower-income sector; Stewart 2004). The legacy of Pinochet's economic model is consequently the division into private and public systems, the former to serve the interests of the high-income group, the latter to take care of the poor and the elderly.[5] The public health system is, furthermore, characterized by insufficient resources, limited services in rural areas, poor and decaying infrastructure, low salaries, lack of medical equipment and medicine and long waiting lists (Borzutsky 2006: 150–151).

MEDICAL PRACTICES AND MENTAL HEALTH IN CHILE

In general, health services are insufficient to deal with demand, particularly in the field of mental health services given the high rate of mental illness in Chile. For instance, a worldwide study of mental health and the prevalence of psychiatric disorders by the World Health Organization (WHO) in 2001 revealed that the figure for depression in Chile is 29.5%, the highest among the countries in the study (see also Han 2012: 25).[6] The prevalence of generalized anxiety was the next highest (18.7%), only surpassed by Brazil (22.6%). In another national study in Chile, 30.1% of women between 25 and 65 reported depressive symptoms within the previous year, while the figure for men was 16% ("Resultado de I encuesta de salud", Chile, Gobierno de Chile, Ministerio de Salud, MINSAL 2003). In addition, a study revealed that 62% of persons who met the criteria for psychiatric disorder did not receive any treatment at all. Of these, 29% responded that they did not know where to go in order to receive assistance. Stigma was also an important barrier to seeking treatment, as a third of the respondents were scared of being diagnosed as mentally ill (Saldivia et al. 2004).

After the transition to democracy in 1990 it was, however, recognized by President Patricio Aylwin that the huge gap between the quality of, and accessibility to, public and private services was a major challenge for the new regime. In consequence, various projects were established, such as the reintroduction of free health services (primary care) and an initiative to build the capabilities of health workers employed therein (Organización

---

[5] There is tendency for women to have less access to the private health system, as only 13.8% of the insured are women (Borzutsky 2006: 152).

[6] According to my own survey, 32% of the respondents claimed to have suffered from depression, 30% from anxiety and 46% from nerves (or *sistema nerviosa*).

Panamericana de la Salud 2002: 85). In 2002 the then president, Ricardo Lagos, launched AUGE (Acesso Universal para Prestaciones Integrales), a plan to improve the public health system. AUGE was to provide coverage for 56 basic diseases (Borzutsky 2006: 152), thereby re-establishing free health services for 3 pathologies, expanded to 40 in 2006; among these were various forms of cancer, diabetes, depression, cardiac problems and schizophrenia (Ministerio de Salud [Minsal] 2006). The field of mental health became a priority of Lagos's government with the establishment of programmes for the treatment of schizophrenia and depression; the latter is recognized as the second largest cause of incapacity or early death.

Thus, as indicated above, public biomedicine in Chile has in many respects failed to meet demand, particularly in the area of mental health. This might be a possible explanation for the widespread use of alternatives, especially Mapuche medicine, in the south of Chile. It is generally acknowledged among medical practitioners that alternative and traditional healing practices commonly provide medical attention for a large group of patients, especially in regard to mental affliction and afflictions not officially recognized as biomedical pathologies. Furthermore, Mapuche treatment is often considered an alternative if the biomedical regimen has been unsuccessful (whether due to lack of access or unsatisfactory diagnosis or treatment).

MAPUCHE MEDICINE: A VALID ALTERNATIVE?

The main practitioners of Mapuche medicine are the machis. Today, with the political recognition of the Mapuche as a people, the machis and Mapuche medicine have entered the political scene, as the machis have been presented as the emblems and guardians of Mapuche culture (Boccara 2002). Although still not officially recognized, Mapuche healing practices and rituals have been granted status as the spiritual essence of the Mapuche, and as fundamental to their continued existence as a people. Paradoxically, Mapuche healers may today practise their medicine due to the Indigenous Law 19.253 of 1993, which guarantees ethnic minorities the right to conserve and develop their own cultural manifestations,[7] but, according to the

---

[7] "El estado reconoce el derecho de los indígenas a mantener y desarollar sus propias manifestationes culturales, en todo lo que no se oponga a la moral, las buenas costumbres y el orden público" (Articulo 7, Ley Indigena 19.253). (The State recognizes indigenous rights to maintain and develop their own cultural manifestation, in ways which do not offend public morals, common customs and the public order. [Indigenous Law 19.253, Articulo 7].)

Sanitary Code, they may still be penalized for practising medicine, although actual lawsuits are rare.[8] Convention OIT 169, ratified in 2009, states that the health system must be organized and administered in collaboration with indigenous peoples (Minsal 2017), but so far this has not led to significant changes (Di Giminiani 2012: 75).

Few statistical accounts exist of the use of Mapuche medicine (Citarella et al. 1995). According to my own survey in Southern Chile, however, it is widespread (as described in Chap. 1). In an urban sector characterized as working class, 90% of those surveyed responded that they had used Mapuche medicine. In a rural area close to the town of Temuco the figure was 95%; in a middle-class area the figure was 40%; while 55% of higher middle-class respondents claimed they had gone to a Mapuche healer. In another study in an urban area, 60% responded that they used both Mapuche healing practices and biomedicine (Torri 2012: 39).

The following account of Mapuche healing practices is primarily based on my own field data, supplemented with local studies. There have been a number of publications on illness and treatment in relation to traditional Mapuche medicine (as noted in Chap. 1), some which are by Chilean anthropologists; these are mainly found in the literature concerning shamanism (Aguirre 2003; Alonqueo 1979; Dowling 1973; Grebe 1972; Foerster 1993; Kuramocho 1991; Montecino 1999). Within Western anthropology, themes such as health, cosmology and rituals among the Mapuche were until recently only discussed in a few exceptional studies such as Lévi-Strauss's work on myths (1968), Mircia Eliade's on shamanism (1964) and in Louis Faron's functionalist-inspired analysis of the social organization of the Mapuche based on fieldwork from 1952 to 1954 (1964, 1968, 1969). The only recent works which take the modern context as a point of departure include a book edited by Citarella et al. (1995) that comprehensively covers the subject of medicine and cultures in the south of Chile, Bacigalupo's work on Mapuche shamans (2001, 2007, 2016a, b, 2018) and Bonelli's work on the Pehuenche (2012, 2014).

According to Bacigalupo (2001), machis were traditionally males, but today 80% are female, although some of the most famous machis in Southern Chile are men. Both male and female machis wear jewellery and

---

[8] An example of a lawsuit is given by the Chilean anthropologist Ana Mariella Bacigalupo, who, in the article "The Mapuche Man Who Became a Woman Shaman", describes the case of a machi who was accused of homicide by poisoning of one of her patients, a 17-year-old boy (Bacigalupo 2004).

coloured scarfs during rituals, when some may also shift genders. For this reason, male machis are often accused of being effeminate (Bacigalupo 2007). Machis are associated with the use of drums (*kultrun*), which they utilize to enter a trance and to invoke spirits and ancestors in ritual and healing practices. The *kultrun* consists of a bowl of laurel or oak filled with stones, corn, seeds and herbal remedies, covered by a skin often depicting symbols that give the particular machi power, such as the moon, stars or thunder. The *kultrun* is conceived of both as a womb and as representing the universe and the corners of the world (*meli wixan mapu*)—north (*pikun*), south (*willi*), east (*puel*) and west (*lafken*).

The machi uses various elements in the healing practice, among these nature, spirits and ancestors as well the deity Ngügechen, which is thought to be present in every aspect of life and death. The deity has four aspects, consisting of a younger and an elderly couple—Old Woman (*kuche*), Old Man (*fucha*), Young Woman (*illcha*) and Young Man (*weche*) (see also Bacigalupo 2007: 50–51). They are connected to the spirit world through their *rewe*, a sacred altar made of a tree trunk often surrounded by canes of colohue and adorned with white, blue or yellow flags and/or the Chilean national flag (Fig. 3.1).

Apart from being health practitioners, the machis also assist in religious Mapuche ceremonies, the most common being *nguillatun*, the fertility ritual. Other Mapuche practitioners exist—*meicas, yerbeteras* and *lawentuchefe*—who do not perform rituals, but mostly treat minor illnesses through the use of herbs; however, the function of ritual expert accords machis great prestige. Neophytes become health practitioners after a period of initiation, often connected to serious illness and spirit visions (*perrimonton*) which are interpreted as a spiritual call (*llamamiento*). The training of a machi normally consists of connecting to the spirit world, with proficiency being demonstrated by the neophyte's increasing expertise in management of the trance state, combined with more factual knowledge of herbs and invocations imparted by one or more initiated machis. On the other hand, some may receive their training from a close family member who is also a machi, without having a *perrimonton*. Generally it is believed that it is only possible to become a machi if two conditions are fulfilled: firstly, the aspirant or his or her family has to own indigenous land; and secondly, it must be established that there are machis within the family lineage, as it is believed that the "spirit of a machi" is transmitted across generations within the same family. The *meicas* or *lawentuchefe* normally diagnose by feeling the pulse of the patient or observing the urine.

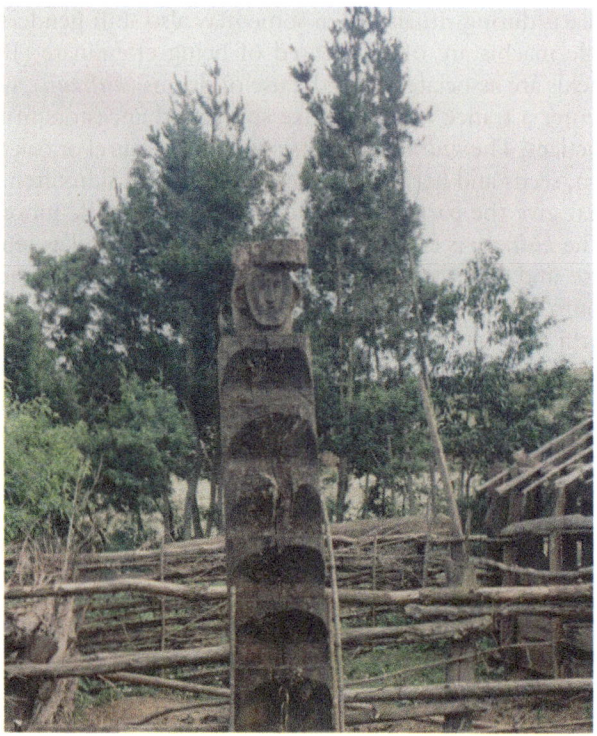

Fig. 3.1   A *rewe*

MAPUCHE ILLNESSES AND MEDICAL PRACTICE

There are different types of illnesses within Mapuche cosmology, a typology that is generally accepted within the Chilean population, categories which have largely integrated biomedical expressions within a range of disease categories.[9] *Re kutran* (natural illnesses) is the term given to those afflictions that are the product of a loss of balance between a person and his or her environment, for instance a sudden shift in temperature or an improper combination of "hot" and "cold" food. Some *re kutran* are regarded as biomedical diseases, such as influenza, colds, wounds, infections, gallstones,

---

[9] These are the most common illnesses which I encountered during my fieldwork. For a more comprehensive list, see Citarella et al. (1995) and Bacigalupo (2007).

tumours and problems related to the eyes and heart. In these types of afflictions patients most often consult a medical doctor or are referred to a medical doctor by a machi, and treatment consists of a combination of
biomedicine with herbal remedies. Other *re kutran* which are most often
treated by Mapuche practitioners are *pasmo*, an affliction produced by a
sudden shift in temperature, the symptoms of which include headache and
eczema, and *empacho*, diarrhoea produced by combining "hot" and "cold"
food or by eating crudely prepared or dirty food; this often affects children.
The treatment consists of herbal remedies and, in the case of *empacho*, in
massaging the coccyx. Another category of diseases, also regarded as *re
kutran*, are *wingka kutran* (foreign illnesses)—thought to have arrived with
the colonizers (*wingka*)—such as tuberculosis, cancer, pneumonia, AIDS
and measles, which are also treated by a medical doctor.

   Then there are the spiritual illnesses, or supernatural illnesses, which
can be subdivided into *wenu kutran*, afflictions caused by deities and spirits, and *weda kutran*, those caused by malign forces. The most common
types of the former are *kastikutran* (punishment illness) and *machikutran*
(shamanic illness). Spirits punish Mapuche with *kastikutran* if they stray
away from traditional norms or fail to fulfil ritual obligations. The most
common types of *weda kutran* are *kalkukutrun*, sickness caused by a witch
(*kalku*), and *wekufetun*, caused by an evil force (wekufe). Lastly there are
also *machikutran*—shamanic illnesses that are accompanied by shamanic
visions (*perrimonton*; Bacigalupo 2007: 31).

   These types of illnesses are not recognized by medical doctors and are
therefore considered the speciality of the machi. As described at the beginning of Chap. 1, symptoms of these types of illnesses include pains (typically in head and stomach, although often they shift location), lack of
energy, dizziness, depression, sadness, weeping, anxiety, lack of appetite,
loss of weight, insomnia and apathy (Bacigalupo 2001: 48–50); these are
similar to those of people diagnosed with depression or anxiety, or what
have been termed the "psychosomatic illnesses of the Chileans" (Agger
and Jensen 1996: 273). In the case of spiritual illness, additional symptoms which were described to me by patients included nightmares and
visions, the feeling of being watched by a strange presence, peculiar sounds
and smells (for instance, what is described as the smell of cemetery soil),
the sudden invasion of maggots, frogs, snakes, insects or vermin into the
house or their appearance in one's food, and being haunted by dogs or
birds, which are thought to be the messengers of evil. Often people feel
that vermin or a lizard (bicho) has entered their body, feeding parasitically

on the body and moving around inside, meaning that the pain likewise moves around.

It is generally believed that people in vulnerable social positions due to poverty, migration or a lack of social networks, as well as those who do not fulfil ritual obligations and fail to observe social norms, are more exposed to illness, especially spiritual illness. Thus, living a balanced life, performing rituals and using antidotes are believed to keep a person free from, or at least less exposed to, spiritual illnesses. If a person is suffering from a spiritual illness, it most commonly affects both physical and social surroundings. The diagnosis of the illness is, however, rarely made on the basis of observed symptoms, even though the set of symptoms described is acknowledged by many people to be an indication of spiritual interference or the harmful actions of human beings. Rather, diagnosis is made by identifying the incident and/or energy that has produced the symptoms, often a spiritual intervention or dramatic event which has caused soul loss (susto). This might take place through dreams (*pewma*) or visions (*perrimonton*) or through an encounter (*trafentun*/susto), where spirits (wekufe) manifest themselves as negative energy, causing illness. Wekufe may have direct encounters with the victims or can appear in dreams and visions (Bacigalupo 2007: 22). Conversely, being possessed by spirits might also be a source of strength and an indication of healing power, depending on how this energy is used and confronted.

Visions frequently involve a *peuchen* (a strange-looking bird), *iwayfilu* (a snake), *witranalwe* (a Spanish horse rider or cowboy demon), *anchimallen* (flying lights which are thought to be the spirits of deceased children who have been bewitched), *cherrufe* (balls of fire) or *meulen* (a strong negative whirling energy). These spirits can be sent by a witch but can also act on their own (*wekufetun*). They often defend an aspect of nature (*ngen*), such as wild forests, marshes and the shores of lakes, lagoons and rivers; if a human being violates their space without permission, it can lead to a temporary loss of soul forces, which manifests itself as a serious illness or deformity (Bacigalupo 2001: 60). It may also jeopardize the normal functioning of both the body and the household, as the spirits cause conflict and loss of self (Bacigalupo 2007: 22). The visions sent by these spirits are best known and most prevalent among the rural Mapuche population, but also occur to some degree among the urban mestizo population in the south.

Another explanation for these symptoms is *kalkutun*; that is, an affliction caused by a witch or a sorcerer who, it is generally believed, may be hired to perform witchcraft (*trabajo*; Bacigalupo 2007: 22). These types of afflictions are called spiritual illnesses—mals (evils) or *daños* (damages)—and are produced in response to envy, jealousy and revenge. To dream about a lizard or an insect might be sign of sorcery (Citarella et al. 1995: 178). Providing the antidote or a *contra* against these acts of sorcery is the speciality of the machi. The most common form of *kalkutun*—and the most common type of affliction among the people who consult the machis—is *infitun*, illness produced by a human agent through the poisoning of beverages, food or objects and considered a possible explanation for symptoms that persist when the medical doctor "cannot find any illness".

Machi treatment involves the use of herbal remedies and ritual, traditionally taking place near the *rewe*, where the machi, by beating a drum (*kultrun*), ritually invoked *ngegechen*, the supreme being, as well as spirits and ancestors. Today, many machis work in urban settings, where they diagnose and give medicine, but they continue to have a *rewe* in their house to which they return in the evening to perform a daily ritual. In cases of natural illness, herbal remedies are usually given and sometimes pharmaceuticals such as aspirins and penicillin; some machis also massage the patient. For spiritual disease, a stronger medicine is required (a *contra*), which usually makes the patient vomit. This latter treatment is often combined with massage, during which the machi extracts objects from the patient's body that are perceived as the evil (mal). The treatment is also combined with the use of *sahumerio*, an exorcism performed by burning herbal remedies accompanied by drumming, in a ritual invocation of spirits (*ulutun*).

When the illness is more serious, a more powerful ritual is performed (*machitun*) in order to expel the evil (mal, wekufe), in which a family member of the patient participates. In the *machitun* the machi enters a trance, during which he or she speaks a ritual language and identifies the cause of the illness and how it can be cured. This information is normally given in the original language of the Mapuche, Mapudungun, which is communicated to the audience by a ritual translator (*dungunmachife*). Machitun is mentioned in early chronicles (Núñez de Pineda 1863: 158–161) and the practices associated with it have in some part remained unaltered, but many machis today incorporate both biomedicine and Christian symbols into their health practices; these can include the use of holy water, the Christian cross and in some cases the invocation of Jesus, the Virgin Mary and Catholic saints (Bacigalupo 2007, 2016a).

As mentioned earlier, however, biomedicine is the only officially valid medical alternative in Chile; therefore, the practice of Mapuche healers is largely influenced by their structural relationship with biomedicine, which is reflected in their adapting of biomedical disease categories to their repertoires. Conversely, medical doctors, although sceptical of Mapuche medicine, often have knowledge of Mapuche illnesses and diagnosis. In the following section the focus is on the diagnostic process, on how patients negotiate the disease categories in the medical systems of biomedicine/psychiatry and shamanistic practice. A central concept here is the medical gaze and the medical knowledge associated with the respective healing system, which is a central element in the construction of personhood.

SCENES FROM MEDICAL PRACTICES: WAYS OF SEEING, KNOWING AND ACTING

In medicine, the authorities who know, the doctors, tend to dominate the known about, the patients. The known about come to behave in the ways that the knowers expect them to. But not always. Sometimes the known about take matters in their own hands. (Hacking 1995: 38)

Philosopher Ian Hacking (1995) writes that disease categories are cultural, social and historical constructions which affect how people experience and manage their bodily conditions as well their understanding of themselves in relation to a social environment, and how they come into being in the first place. This forms part of a dynamic process which Hacking designates "making up people", which takes place in the relationship between "people who are known about, the knowledge about them, and the knowers" (Hacking 1995: 6). Thus, a bodily experience is mediated and formed by the practitioner and the disease categories that are available in a given social context for articulating and experiencing bodily and psychological distress.

In the following I examine the diagnostic process and its social implications for the illness experience of the patients. The analytical focus is on the medical gaze—that is, the "construction" of the eyes that see the disease category—in biomedicine/psychiatry and Mapuche medicine/shamanistic healing (Foucault 1994 [1973]). In the *Birth of the Clinic* (1973), Foucault explores how medical knowledge and practice produce a certain body, thereby establishing medical power at a micro level. He describes the historical development of the modern medical gaze; that is, the trained eye of medical professionals, who possess the knowledge to read the symptoms and signs of a disease. In the medical gaze the human body becomes the sum of a person, and the trained medical eye knows how to observe the signs and symptoms that correspond to a disease category, be it of a biological or psychological nature. The symptom is the form in which the disease is presented; it allows the invariable nature of the disease to show through (Foucault 1973: 90). The medical professional has been trained to observe and "read" the signs and symptoms, which implies a distancing from the subjective experience of the patient.

Under the medical gaze—comprising the medical practitioners' perceptions and experiences—a person's "constitution" can be read through an array of signs. Based on diagnostic criteria, the aim is to decide whether a patient's symptoms correspond to a "real" biomedical category. The mind/body dualism is fundamental to this, meaning that some diseases are granted the status of "real" biological and categorical entities, while others are considered conditions of the mind. However, the latter are still considered disease categories to be discerned through observing and seeing the patient with a trained medical gaze. The doctor becomes a sort of miracle worker who knows how to read the signs of the body; she or he is the authority, aiming to establish reason in the mind of the patient. Medical practice therefore has a strong moral function as the regulating force over human behaviour and "inner" thoughts, and forms part of a broader apparatus of moral control in society. In his volumes on sexuality (1979), Foucault calls this regulating force "biopower".

The medical gaze of shamanistic (machi) practice is of a fundamentally different character: first and foremost the shaman does not only observe the patient who is present, she or he also sees into past and future times, and senses through touching (the pulse and clothes). According to Mapuche cosmology there is no separation between mind and body, nor between the individual and the social body. Moreover, in shamanistic practice the body is not considered to be a closed system; rather, the individual body is regarded as an open entity connected to and influenced by external social and spiritual forces and susceptible to moral acts. Illness is regarded as a consequence of a loss of balance, for instance an improper balance in food or temperature. An illness is thought to affect the spiritual, physical and social aspects of a person's being; in other words, emotions, physical organs and social relations are all interdependent. Consequently, it is believed that an occurrence in a person's present (or past) may affect his or her own well-being, as well as the well-being of those with whom she or he is connected socially (Grebe 1972; Bacigalupo 2001: 42; Citarella et al. 1995). Moreover, it is believed that numinous powers make their presence felt through signs that must be interpreted if one is to understand the meaning of life. Therefore, the "signs" and "symptoms" do not correspond to a categorical disease entity; rather, they refer to social disorders and imbalances in the relationship between a patient and his or her social environment caused by soul loss, social conflict or witchcraft (Bacigalupo 2007: 25–29).

As there are no fixed disease categories in shamanistic practice, illness becomes a social phenomenon, since it is thought to affect the patient's social environment. As such, the "sign" for seeing and identifying the illness is not only the work of the practitioner, but is also in the hands of the patient and the "therapy management group" (defined by John Janzen as consisting of "kinsmen and friends, who are mobilized when illness strikes an individual and which acts to define the situation and to search for a remedy" [1978: xi]). This "fragmenting" of fixed disease categories moves the patient into an intersubjective and shared world of illness experiences. Meanwhile, given that the public health setting is characterized by limited resources, patients have the opportunity to address their illness symptoms within an arena of medical pluralism. This has far-reaching social implications for relations between patient and practitioner, which I explore in what follows via scenes of interaction between patients and practitioners during the process of diagnosis, especially those involving the therapy management group, in the process of locating and identifying illness.

The gaze in medical practice serves to construct certain notions of a human being by providing a language through which patients shape their understanding of, and interaction with, their social world. Western disease categories—in this case a psychoanalytic model of a separation between mind and body, conscious and unconscious—have served as the model for classifying symptoms in biomedical practice wherein a disease has either an organic cause, or is expected to "fit" categories of mental disease, as stated in the diagnostic manuals of mental disorders (DSM IV or ICT10). When health problems do not fit disease categories—with so-called medically unexplained symptoms (Kirmayer 2004), such as somatic complaints without an organic pathology, or very "unusual" expressions of mental disease— adjustments have been made, producing the diagnoses of somatization or psychosomatic disorders (Kleinman 1986; see Chap. 1). In contrast, the disease categories in shamanistic practice are of a fundamentally different nature, which leads to different social implications for the relationship between patient and practitioner and the patient's negotiation of his or her social position. Indeed, by making the medical choice to pursue shamanistic treatment, the patient not only enters an intersubjective world of shared understanding, but also articulates a basic distrust of the public health setting and/or biomedical system.

It is, however, crucial to stress that the end result is not necessarily a choice between a biomedical or a shamanistic disease category; rather, it is more likely to be combination of the two different medical fields. In that sense the medical scenes presented in the following section are not seen as exclusive, but as parallel options in the patient's medical choices. One might even suggest that being sick often reflects a strategic choice. Both biomedical and shamanistic categories appeal to patients, but for different reasons and as part of different sets of strategies. It is precisely in the interaction *between* the medical systems in a specific context that patients negotiate their position through experiences of dissonance or resonance between life experiences and medical practice. Thus, what might seem like opposed regimes of diagnosis are in fact complementary in the medical choices of patients. This point is explored in the following section in order to understand the diagnostic process, and later in connection with medical dialogue (in Chap. 4) and bodily symptoms (Chap. 5). Moreover, later it will be explored how themes of cultural repression—olvidos as divisions based on class and ethnicity, as well as experiences of terror, violence and vulnerability—emerge and are transformed through the use of Mapuche medicine. In the following the field setting will be described, with a focus on the actual medical procedures of the health practitioner.

IMAGINED MALADIES: "DISEASES OF THE HEAD"

We have a problem here which I would call the law of minor efforts. The people just love medical certificates,[10] because they do not like to work, and in order not to work they become ill. They start to produce physical symptoms, and they go to a psychiatrist; they start crying, they feel dizzy and claim that the end of the world has arrived and that they are going to die. Then the psychiatrist gives them a medical certificate, 15 days, 20 days, then a month, along with the message, "Go home and relax." Honestly, I believe that there is a great deal of theatrical performance and simulation of the state of things. The majority of the people in this country are not sick. If you begin to analyse the greater majority of medical consultations, they are

---

[10] A medical certificate is an official document that is issued by clinicians and required in order for students and workers to be excused from school or work responsibilities and to lay claim to such things as disability payments.

mostly psychiatric consultations with the motive of acquiring medical certificates, due to depressions, anxieties related to specific occurrences, problems
with the husband or the kids or problems at the workplace. All this starts to
accumulate. Then people start to seek solutions in the medical system and
end up with a medical certificate. This is our own way of doing things, our
mentality.

This is how a Chilean physician at the Hospital Regional de Temuco characterizes the health condition of the majority of his patients. In a similar
vein, one of his colleagues (quoted in Chap. 1) estimates that in approximately 70% of medical consultations no organic pathology can be detected.
In other words, the patients have no "real" disease; rather, their symptoms—including aches and pains—have a purely psychological and social
origin. The physician claims that the patients suffer from "imagined" illnesses which often serve non-medical purposes like getting increased
attention and being liberated from work responsibilities, in the workplace
as well as the home.

Chilean patients challenge the system of knowledge of biomedical doctors, as the symptoms and signs displayed by many patients often fail to
correspond to biological disease categories; that is, most patients do not
suffer from any organic pathology observable with a trained medical gaze.
The doctor quoted above recognized the widespread use of placebos:
"These afflictions can be treated with placebos; they need time to work,
and they need a magical treatment. Yes, we doctors also know how to perform magic, in the same way as the Mapuche."[11] By providing a diagnosis
and a placebo, doctors forestall patients' seeking of another practitioner. As
the same doctor put it, "We know that the patient will continue to go from
practitioner to practitioner until one says, 'This is what you have; take this
and you'll be fine.'" In a similar vein, Dr Silva, head of the Department of
Medicine at a university in Temuco, admonishes his students never to tell
a patient that nothing is wrong. He points out that the three most important events of a consultation are examination, followed by a diagnosis and,
lastly, medication. If there is nothing wrong with the patient, she or he
must be given a placebo, which apparently happens in many cases.

A vast majority of the patients in the general practitioners' clinics are
diagnosed as suffering from afflictions characterized as non-organic, such
as depression, anxiety or problems related to the nervous system (*sistema
nerviosa*). The patients' own category is that of nervios, which refers to an

[11] Interview with Dr Eduardo Paez.

illness with physical, emotional and spiritual components that is common in Latin America. Many who experience nervios feel out of control and alien in their bodies (Bacigalupo 2007: 72). The condition may be produced by a breakdown in the family network and concern about the well-being of kin and family (Low 1994). To the doctors, nervios is largely perceived as psychosomatic and caused by social distress or, as one doctor said to a patient, "There is nothing wrong with you, your problem is only in here," pointing to the patient's head. Those with abdominal pains are often diagnosed with irritable bowel syndrome, also a condition that, although characterized by pain, is not a "real" organic pathology, but a syndrome related to social stress (Kirmayer 1988).

As the preceding section shows, a dichotomy is put in place between "real diseases", the ones where an organic pathology can be revealed, and "imagined" diseases, the ones "in the head". All are given a diagnosis and medicine; however, the "biological" is considered more "real". When no organic pathology is detected, symptoms are considered the preserve of the specialists of "imagined maladies" and "diseases of the head", the psychologists, neurologists and psychologists; to these practitioners "diseases of the head" do have validity as "real" categories. When no biological diagnosis can be offered, many patients accept a psychiatric diagnosis. Dr Silva is an expert in the latter and deals with many such cases in his clinic in Temuco's local hospital, the Hospital Regional Hernán Henriquez Aravena.[12] Several doctors at the hospital participated in the study; however, as mentioned in Chap. 1, only Dr Silva—head of the Department of Psychiatry, Psychology and Neurology at the hospital—was involved on a more regular basis. The cost of a consultation at the hospital is covered by health insurance (FONASA/ISAPRES).

SCENES FROM A PSYCHIATRIST'S WAITING ROOM IN A PUBLIC HEALTH SETTING

The first sight that greets visitors and patients in the polyclinic for psychiatry, psychology and neurology is the huge number of people waiting: in the small waiting room, in the corridors. The supply of appointments does

---

[12] In 1929 the construction of the Hospital Regional Temuco commenced; it was completed in 1933. In 1976 it was remodelled to its current design and in 2004 was renamed the Hospital Regional Hernán Henriquez Aravena. Today the hospital also functions as a university hospital and forms part of the Faculdad de Medicina de la Universidad de la Frontera as an institution for higher education.

not begin to meet the demand. If patients have managed to get an appointment at all, they are all scheduled for 9:30 a.m. Normally they turn up at least two hours early to be sure not to miss the appointment.

Dr Silva's clinic is located in a basement, where approximately 30–40 patients are waiting for the consultation hour to start. The decoration is sparse and includes a Mapuche calendar with a picture of the machi Sebastian, and a sign saying that there are no more appointments available for infant psychiatry until further notice. Alongside this a wag has written, in a childish scribble, "Why doesn't the consultant psychiatrist take care of them; that is what he is paid to do." Normally, around half of the patients are waiting for Dr Silva and others for other specialities. Two ladies in white coats behind a desk register the patients as they arrive and call out the name of the next patient. Most patients have a Mapuche surname. This is hardly surprising, as the public health setting is meant for the lower strata of Chilean society, to which most people who identify as indigenous belong.

The atmosphere in the waiting room is quite tense and people are taciturn; no one comments openly on their reason for being there. Someone makes a remark about the long wait; another person comments that people stay overnight to get appointments with specialists. I often spend around an hour and a half waiting in almost complete silence, as Dr Silva gives me the same appointment time as his patients, 9:30 a.m., but rarely shows up before 11. I try to make contact with people by asking questions like "Where are you from?", which normally opens a conversation in any public room; in this setting people just give me monosyllabic replies. I see a man I have met on another occasion, but he seems very uncomfortable on meeting me here and hardly greets me. His wife tells me that he has been treated for depression but has stopped the treatment; now they are back again, because he is "quite bad". A woman beside him says that often the medicine does not help much. The wife comments that it does help some, but of course not completely. Another time I happen to run into a neighbour. I ask her why she is here; she tells me in a low voice that she is being treated for depression, but also needs to renew her medical certificate.[13] I am surprised to meet her here, as she has only mentioned visits to machis and herbalists in our earlier conversations. She quickly moves on and I do not get the chance to discover more. These incidents show that

---

[13] When I later run into her on the street, she explains to me that she needed the medical certificate for a grant application for her daughter's university studies.

psychiatric treatment is, to a large degree, stigmatizing, so that people feel that others will be suspicious if they hear that they are being treated by a psychiatrist, that they will be accused of being "mad".

Another conspicuous feature in this setting is the pervasive presence of Mapuche culture. I talk to the social worker, who has an office opposite Dr Silva's clinic. She is very sweet and kind and offers me a chair, but claims to be "extremely" busy. We are interrupted by a poor-looking Mapuche woman, who comes into the office to thank the psychiatric staff for having completely cured her daughter of her "madness". "You see," she tells me, "my daughter became disturbed, because she was bewitched with something someone had put into the water." When she leaves I ask the social worker why the woman had not seen a machi if she believed that the madness was caused by witchcraft. "Probably she has," the social worker says. "They all consult the machi." She adds that she "likes Mapuche culture and rituals a lot," then she turns back to the papers in front of her. I start talking about what I know of different machis in the area, and her interest in me suddenly increases. "Oh," she says, "perhaps you could recommend a machi to me; I have so many health problems which I need to solve." I promise to give her a list of the machis I know and she seems very grateful.

Scenes from a Psychiatric Consultation

After hours of waiting Dr Silva appears, and invites me in a friendly way into his consulting room, which has a chair on one side for the practitioner, two for patients, and a brown couch where I take a seat together with a medical student. Along the wall is a table with a calendar, a telephone and a model of a ship; on his desk a pile of case records. Dr Silva opens a case record, gives us the name of the patient, the age and current diagnosis, medicines prescribed and progress of treatment, then calls the patient. The following consultation is selected as being quite typical, involving the most common type of patient in Chilean medical practice: a woman aged between 20 and 65, suffering from depression (Ministerio de Salud 1998).

Describing the patient, Dr Silva says, "Maria is an evangelic priest with severe depression, which has been very difficult to treat. She has been prescribed an antidepressant, which she takes." A lady with red hair, slightly overweight, about 40 years old, comes in with her husband. She walks slowly and has a very troubled expression on her face. She sits down with her husband and the consultation starts.

Dr Silva:	I am sorry you had to wait so long. Is there any change?
Maria:	The accumulation inside continues [she breathes heavily], nothing seems to bring me pleasure. I feel a great pressure here [points at her chest]. Sometimes I only want to cry.
Dr Silva:	Have you been able to participate in any social activities?
Maria:	It is as though something prevents me; my mind is as frozen [she smiles resignedly].
Dr Silva:	But I notice a difference. Apparently I just saw you smile.
Maria:	When I am outside people say that I am not sick, and I have to explain to them that it is something inside me.
Dr Silva:	But your facial expression is less troubled. [He turns to the husband.] I want to know how you see her, your wife.
Husband:	I have faith that she will recover; she is not crying as much as before. I have noticed a change.
Dr Silva:	For how many days has she taken 50 ml?
Husband:	Fourteen days.
Dr Silva:	Then some change must have occurred.
Maria:	If only I could get rid of this thing inside here. [She points at her chest again and smiles.]
Dr Silva:	I do not know if you agree with me?
Husband:	Yes, she did smile.
Dr Silva:	A quick-acting anti-depressant doesn't exist. She has to take it for at least 21 days before it really starts to be effective. Now she must start taking 50 ml twice a day. [He gives her the medicine.]
Husband:	But things have improved at home, our children have started to help their mother much more.
Dr Silva:	That is fine.

In this exchange, the validity of the diagnosis was not in question, although Maria apparently had problems in getting her social world to recognize her depression. Dr Silva, Maria and her husband had all accepted the diagnosis of depression as a valid description of her state. Maria's symptoms did correspond to those listed in a manual for the diagnosis and treatment of depression produced by the Ministry of Health (Ministerio de Salud 1998: 31), wherein the three most common are listed as tiredness, sadness and a lack of interest and participation in social activities.[14] Dr Silva's

---

[14] The two most important questions for diagnosing depression according to CIE 10 are listed as "¿Se ha sentido triste o deprimida la mayor parte del tiempo, o casi todos los días?"

question about participation in social activities was posed to establish whether the symptoms were present and to see if the prescribed medicine had produced an effect, the same reason as he had involved Maria's husband. Maria also complained of pain in the chest. In the manual, as in Silva's diagnosis, these are not regarded as "real" physical symptoms, but as a sign of the patient's psychological state, arising because the patient does not recognize her psychological condition but, rather, lives it somatically. Dr Silva explained to me that this kind of depression is called a "masked" depression and often occurs among the Mapuche and patients from the lower social strata. Dr Silva is the professional medical authority who, with a trained medical gaze, knows how to evaluate the symptoms of the patient according to a checklist to establish a disease category, in this case depression. He perceives the illness as a biomedically defined category with a fixed list of symptoms, meanwhile also recognizing the importance of social relations in its treatment.

In the next medical exchange, with Gabriella, Dr Silva's role is not confined to "reading" the signs and symptoms of a disease category, but extends to "helping" the patient to sift reason from unreason. Gabriella is a slim, middle-aged woman with a high-pitched, very nervous voice, which constantly breaks with emotion.

Dr Silva: What has happened?
Gabriella: Do you know, doctor, I feel so terrible. I work with a photocopier in order to pay for my son's university. I borrowed money to pay for it, but still I cannot pay. I really do not know how to manage, and he only has four more exams.
Dr Silva: And where does he study?
Gabriella: At the Mayor [a local private university]. I went to see them and they told me that I could pay 160,000 pesos [around 200 euros] in four instalments. I started to work with the photocopier, but I feel a strange presence, and toads surround my house.
Dr Silva: Did you all see them [the toads and strange presences]?
Gabriella: Yes, we all saw them. And now I cannot concentrate on taking photocopies. I feel anxious, as though something is haunting me, when I open the door it is like…

and "¿Ha estado desinteresada (o) o incapaz de disfrutar la vida la mayor parte del tiempo, casi todos los días?" (Ministerio de Salud 1998).

Dr Silva:	Like expecting bad news?
Gabriella:	Yes.
Dr Silva:	And this presence, is it not something you have invented yourself?
Gabriella:	No, doctor, I felt that something fell down on the ground.
Dr Silva:	And didn't you have someone to cleanse the house?
Gabriella:	Some people have recommended a witch with lots of power, because this is something really strong.
Dr Silva:	And what does your husband think about this?
Gabriella:	I told all this to a parapsychologist from Santiago, but I am not sure about it. My husband feels the same about it as I do. Do you know one day we found a lizard beneath the cooker. It is as though suddenly… [she is interrupted by Dr Silva].
Dr Silva:	And what about your daughter, does she know about it?
Gabriella:	I have not told her what is happening. But my husband knows; he also saw the witchcraft, he saw evil animals, stains. I went to the university in order to talk to the headmaster about the situation.
Dr Silva:	And your son is not studying?
Gabriella:	At the moment he is not studying. There are so many things that you can only tell a professional. Doctor, I need a medical certificate to present at the university.
Dr Silva:	Don't worry, we will give you one.

Dr Silva gives her a prescription for tranquillizers; she thanks him and leaves rapidly. After Gabriella has left, Dr Silva explains to me (and to the medical student present) that she thinks she has been a victim of witchcraft, of which the insects and reptiles are signs. Dr Silva is familiar with the "animistic" world in which most of his patients live; however, he diagnoses her as "suffering from hallucinations, also called paranoia". His integration of the opinions of other family members was, he explains, to observe whether they shared the hallucination, adding, "They all live the same fantasy in a world full of magic and signals." He also diagnosed the woman as suffering from "psychological disturbance" and "severe depression", signified by her sadness and anxiety, and explained that he identified states of anxiety if a patient answered in the affirmative when asked whether she is "expecting bad news"; an affirmative also reveals hallucinations. He tried to make Gabriella see reason by suggesting that she might have invented the hallucination herself; the denial of this became a sign of "psychological disturbance".

THE MEDICAL PRACTICE OF THE PSYCHIATRIST: THE BIO-PSYCHO-SOCIAL GAZE

Although both Maria and Gabriella had experienced symptoms and problems that were not strictly mental (in Maria's case, the pain in the chest; in Gabriella's, things entering the house), their diagnosis located their problems "in the mind", invoking depression and a state of anxiety corresponding to "the intrapsychic" or "psychosocial" models described in Chap. 1. The physical symptoms (Maria's pain) and the occurrences in Gabriella's house were both regarded as products of psychological disturbance. This corresponds to the medical ideology that if no organic cause can be observed, the problem is located in the mind. The observing psychiatrist poses a sequence of questions that are standardized in order to identify the category suitable for diagnosis and treatment. The medical consultation serves to identify a predetermined set of symptoms that fit already-defined disease categories. Individual diseases are considered natural categories that are not dependent on social interaction and subjective experiences. The symptoms are the signs, which only the doctor, the medical authority, knows how to read. The symptoms reveal the disease. Here some combinations of symptoms are considered to reveal the diagnosis directly (sadness, lack of energy and tiredness might indicate depression, for instance). Thus, the diagnosis was not only an instrument for observing disease, but also the instrument of a moral apparatus that sets up standards for sane/insane, healthy/unhealthy. However, the diagnosis actually became an official recognition of their symptoms, which served a certain strategic aim.

In these scenes the prime aim was not to identify the cause of the depression, but rather to treat the symptoms. However, Dr Silva, like the other staff I interviewed, acknowledged the role of social and psychological factors; among these were mentioned family disputes, economic problems, unemployment, violence, alcohol dependency, migration and lack of social support. Recognizing the limited resources at his disposal, however, he said that he could only treat people's symptoms, not help them live their lives. While such explanations were not rejected, they did not play any major role in the actual medical treatment beyond the recognition of the role of social relations in mental health, which resulted in Dr Silva's attempt to involve the patient's close social relations in treatment of the affliction. Therefore, as described, Dr Silva's medical practice and diagnosis became a resource and a strategy in the patients' social lives. In Maria's case, the diagnosis of depression might have helped to get her social network to acknowledge her illness, while Gabriella's medical certificate probably helped her to negotiate her debt with the university.

The hospital would not grant me permission to interview patients later, away from the hospital, so I have no indication of how Maria and Gabriella perceived the diagnosis and treatment provided by Dr Silva. In order to explore this question, the focus in the following is on another patient, Sonia, who consulted a shaman (machi José Caripan) with similar symptoms as those described in the psychiatrist's consultation—that is, pain in chest, sadness and "magical" occurrences—and had a medical diagnosis of depression and "nerves". Her story offers a key to understanding the social and collective dynamics related to the diagnostic process; that is, how it affects a patient's relationship to the practitioner and her social connections. The notion of disease categories is fundamentally different in shamanistic practice as, unlike in biomedicine, diagnoses are not formalized. This means that the work of diagnosis and the reading of "signs" and "symptoms" is not aimed at identifying an established disease category, but rather their cause, mostly perceived as an imbalance between a person and his or her environment. The patients and their relatives might also be involved in identifying and establishing the cause, which makes the process of diagnosis fundamentally different. Furthermore, I propose that the key to understanding the effectiveness of shamanistic practice is to utilize not only an intrapsychic model of illness, but also a sociosomatic model where the focus is on the relationship between illness experience, medical practice and socio-political reality (as described in Chap. 1); that is, illness is connected not only to individual distress, but also to collective experiences of suffering. In other words, the diagnostic process becomes embedded in social relations and part of the process of making personhood. Meanwhile, the way the women present their sickness is linked to their articulating and negotiating their social positioning. In the cases of Gabriella and Maria, the gains were obvious: for Maria, increased attention and decreased domestic responsibility; and for Gabriella, a medical certificate which helped her in her struggle to resolve the debt with the university. However, by using multiple medical choices the patients' range of agency is expanded. Sonia's story is an example of this.

While I did not have the chance to interview either Maria or Gabriella, I did interview a number of patients, Sonia among them, who had been treated for depression by a physician and/or psychiatrist. Their accounts of treatment were quite similar. Although the diagnosis of depression or anxiety covered a range of symptoms (lack of energy, desire to cry, desire to die), people said that it did not explain their physical pains or their more "spiritual" experiences. Many, however, accepted the diagnosis as valid, treating their depression with medicine, combined, in some cases, with psychological help. On the other hand, respondents reported that they could not reveal all their symptoms to the medical doctors, and nor did the latter have time to listen to them; it was further claimed that the medicine received for depression brought relief for a short period but, although it might have stopped them from "crying too much", it never really affected "the root of the problem". Several of the patients had received psychological counselling and one woman said it had helped her control her depression and bodily pain, but it never really "explained anything". Two people commented that "at the psychologist they did nothing more than talk", and that it did not really help as they were not "given any medicine". The diagnosis and treatment through both psychiatry and shamanistic medicine apparently had a much more profound impact, explored below, where we see that biomedicine provided an official recognition of symptoms, while shamanistic practice involved social relations in the identification of the cause of the illness. Hence the two types of medicine served different strategic aims.

In other words, what people were seeking through multiple medical choices can be summed up in three words: diagnosis, explanation and medicine. They appeared to feel that this would make the bodily state tangible and open up possibilities for acting, but only if they (the patients) received what they regarded as a "real" diagnosis. Patients requested different types of medicine, and used them simultaneously, in a parallel way, but the diagnostic processes involved in procuring them differed, particularly in connection with the relationship between "real" and "non-real" diagnosis and the interaction between patient, practitioner and therapy management group. As one woman commented about her treatment with both her general practitioner and a psychologist:

> I did not know what I was fighting against. It is awful not having a diagnosis. It is much easier knowing, for instance, I have cancer: now I have a cancer and I have to do this and that. But without a "real" diagnosis, when they say that there is nothing wrong with you, or that it is "just" your nerves, that leaves you without any possibilities for acting.

In the following section I explore Sonia's illness story and consultation at a shaman's house. She had been treated by both a medical doctor and a psychologist for depression and nerves; however, she did not consider these "real" sickness categories, thereby reproducing the biomedical version of biological sickness as a "real" category. Just like the other patients, Sonia too was searching for a "real" diagnosis (that is, not a psychiatric category), and only turned to shamanistic medical practice because her biomedical doctor could not provide her with a diagnosis which she found broad enough to cover all symptoms, psychological, physiological and spiritual.

SCENES FROM A SHAMAN'S WAITING ROOM

As we shall see, the diagnostic process at the shaman's house is very much embedded in dialogues that take place in the waiting room. I explore these in order to show the central role that the community of patients plays in the process of getting a diagnosis. During fieldwork I attended healing and diagnosis sessions in the house of José Caripan, a shaman in his 50s, who lived with his family (wife and two daughters) near a tourist centre, about 80 miles from Temuco. Twice a week he attended patients at his private house, where he had constructed two waiting rooms and a consultation room.

The patients bring a bottle containing their urine, labelled with their name and age, which they leave in a separate building that serves as the "consultation room" and "office"; some also bring urine from family members, friends or neighbours. Then the shaman examines the bottles in turn; he explained to me that he could see the bodies of the patients reflected in the urine and he then received messages from his spiritual helpers. He integrates collective rituals in the morning and evening into his medical practice, performing a healing ritual at 8 a.m. during which he sings, plays his drum and calls upon nature spirits and the Virgin of Carmen, the national saint of Chile. As a spiritual authority who is connected to divine power, the shaman is a messenger with the gift to channel communications from another reality. Through his ritual, José purifies the crowd with holy water and incense, turning the scene into a combination of a Mapuche ceremony and a Catholic mass. Afterwards, he returns to his ongoing work of diagnosis.

While I had many difficulties furthering contact with patients going to Dr Silva, staying at José's house made this easy. People arrived prepared to "hang out", bringing their own coffee and picnic basket or buying food and drinks there, and had organized themselves so they could stay all day, some even staying on after they had received their medicine. During the many hours they spent there, people would share illness narratives, many of which contained strong criticism of biomedical doctors, of how they only practise medicine in order to get rich. Some commented that doctors do not accept symptoms that do not fit their already-established categories, making the patient seem foolish. The narratives also revealed ideas and experiences which the doctors "would never accept" and which "could not be shared openly", namely, the experiences of being ill due to humoural imbalances (*pasmo*), the evil eye (*mal ojo*) or damage brought about by external agents in response to moral transgression (mal/susto). Bodily experiences and feelings of "strange" presences and occurrences were widely narrated and shared among the patients, as well as stories of how good and evil forces intrude on and affect human existence. These are experiences that almost everyone shares, and if a patient does not already know the terminology, this setting is the perfect way to get insight into it and find out whether one's own symptoms fit an indigenous or popular category of illness. Often newcomers would be comforted with comments like "He can solve your problem, do not worry, you are not alone."

SCENE FROM A SHAMAN'S CONSULTATION: SONIA

I met Sonia, a 38-year-old woman who identified herself as mestizo, early one morning when she was travelling to José's house by bus, along with her mother. Sonia worked in a kindergarten in a Mapuche reservation, some distance from José, where she lived with her husband and her 20-year-old daughter. The husband worked as a nursing auxiliary in a public health clinic. Sonia claimed to be content with her life among the Mapuche, getting along really well with the people there. However, her mother once commented to me that when Sonia married at the age of 17 and moved to her husband's place on the reservation, she was so sad that that the mother had to move in with her to comfort her.

The first time I met her, Sonia was staying with her mother, who lived near José's house, during the summer vacation. This gave her the opportunity to consult the shaman. Mother and daughter looked very alike: both had smiling faces and short, dyed-blonde hair. In the bus they chattered in a lively fashion, but also seemed quite tense. When they arrived at José's house I noticed that they waited impatiently for hours for their turn, as the place was especially packed with people that day. When José finally asked Sonia to come up and receive her diagnosis, he was very sinister, almost shouting at her without giving her a chance to answer. "You have a great evil!" he said, without explaining what it was; he continued,

"You imagine yourself lying in a coffin. You must not think like this, because you have a family and must stay alive." Then he explained that she had a problem with too much liquid in her heart, which could be treated with his medicine. It was a very dramatic moment, as Sonia started crying almost hysterically while her mother tried to comfort her.

How should we characterize this shamanistic medical gaze compared with Dr Silva's? In a sense, Sonia's reaction might fit Freud's descriptions of the hysterical women of Vienna who had no outlet for their psychological and sexual frustrations. Or could it be seen as corresponding to Dr Silva's description of a "masked" depression; that is, a depression characterized by somatic complaints without a "real" basis, an organic explanation? On the other hand, as demonstrated in the following section, José's diagnosis acknowledged the somatic complaints as "real". Furthermore, rather than merely identifying the signs—sadness, lack of appetite, lack of energy, insomnia—which could be an indication of a disease category such as depression, José's diagnosis had the distinction of discerning the need for a response that encompassed and addressed the full spectrum of Sonia's psychological and physical condition. This broke her social isolation and triggered an intense emotional reaction; it also influenced her affliction.

Diagnostic and Social Processes

I visited Sonia at her mother's place on several occasions after her session with José. Her mother lived alone with a grandchild, the daughter of Sonia's sister, who worked as a household help in Santiago. Both Sonia and her sister spent the summer with their daughters at their mother's house, where they discussed, among other topics, many health issues, now especially Sonia's "great evil". As we were having wonderful summer weather and Sonia's mother lived near the beach, I remarked that they must be having a good time. I was quite surprised to hear that in the past two months they had been out of the house only once, other than the visit to José, as they did not like "people" and did not like "going out".

This lack of social life was explained by Sonia's "illness". Sonia had suffered from intense pains in the head and heart and from a depressive mood for many years. She had no energy, no desire to get up in the morning. She hardly slept at night, often felt dizzy and nauseous, and often wished she could stop living. She had undergone numerous medical examinations, which revealed no organic problems, and a medical doctor had consequently diagnosed her as suffering from a disorder of the nervous system.

Sonia revealed that she was very disappointed in medical doctors; they never cured her, merely making her feel ashamed by suggesting that she was not "really ill" and only suffering "from nerves". At some point her daughter, who was studying to be a medical secretary, suggested that her mother might have depression. Sonia went to a doctor, who confirmed the diagnosis and gave her medicine, but the medicine made her feel awful: she started shaking and would on occasion lose her memory; for instance, she would suddenly feel she was lost, even in a familiar place, forgetting where and with whom she was.

Apart from thinking that her mother was depressive, the daughter also suggested that a Mapuche woman, who was interested in her father, had bewitched her. This might be "the evil" to which José had referred. The daughter complained that her mother showed "too much confidence" in drinking *mate* (a local caffeine-rich infusion) with the Mapuche. This made her vulnerable to attempted attack by witchcraft. Sonia's mother supported this idea, saying that it was confirmed by the many stories of witchcraft shared at José's house.

In the beginning Sonia believed that "the great evil" referred to the heart condition and the problem with "too much liquid". However, later she told me of a vision she had had of a dark-skinned boy who showed up and then suddenly disappeared; she thought that this might be an omen indicating that evil forces were at work. She then told me about finding an old book on witchcraft at her workplace that confirmed the suspicion; moreover, she said, she had bought a cheese from a Mapuche woman, which turned out to be full of worms even though it was completely fresh. She immediately burned the cheese; this produced such a bad smell that the neighbours commented on it—it was definitely not a normal cheese. Finally, she told me about how the local church had burnt down; this was such a dramatic incident that after it her condition worsened. On some days she even had to leave work due to nervous attacks and sudden loss of memory.

José's diagnosis, however, became a turning point. At first she had felt overwhelmed and very upset, but had simultaneously experienced the incredible relief of meeting someone who understood and saw her sufferings. After taking the medicine he provided she instantly felt better, stopped worrying, started sleeping and felt alive again. So eager was she to get well, she drank all the medicine in four days, afterwards returning to her depressive mood. Sonia's biggest worry was how to procure the medicine after going home. Her mother jokingly said that the best solution was to take the shaman with her, so he could continue to make it for her; however, Sonia thought that she could take some time off and visit him again.

To me, it was interesting to know that although Sonia's family considered themselves Chilean, or non-indigenous, they all had a strong belief in the power of Mapuche medicine; they said that the Mapuche know how to cure, but also how to harm. Sonia herself was very positive, observing that the shaman treated her as a person; "He takes people seriously, sees them as human beings rather than as objects," she said. She and her family agreed that "the shaman really knows the secrets of nature, it is spiritual heritage, not only a result of studying books". She expressed gratitude towards José for being able to see her problems, which led her to trust his medicine and also gave her back her trust in life. In contrast, Sonia and her family said that "doctors would leave you dying outside the hospital if you cannot give them a cheque of guarantee". Sonia's sister also told me that she once almost underwent surgery for breast cancer, when another examination by another doctor revealed that she did not have cancer at all. "They invent illnesses and ask for tests just to make you nervous and to get money out of you," she complained, "and it does not help to sue them; as poor people we could never win." They all agreed that they find it hard to take any practitioner seriously who is not Mapuche. Later Sonia went back to José with the hope of learning more about her "evil", but again she returned without a clear answer. She continued to be divided between the explanation of witchcraft and the possibility that "the great evil" referred to her heart condition. But she never doubted that José had the answer. Sonia's quest for therapy has not ended here, and she will probably return to José or another shaman, as most of my other informants did, thereby transforming traditional healing into an integral part of daily existence.

Thus, there is no proper conclusion to Sonia's story. As often happens, the consultation at José's gave Sonia some relief and, more particularly, it gave her a sense of meaning, coherence and security, as well as a possible language for articulating her distress and for acting against it. Consequently, Lévi-Strauss's idea of shamanistic practice as useful for providing a language for expressing distress is, in Sonia's case, of some relevance. But is the effectiveness of medicine then connected to the patient's rational understanding and her recovery of meaningfulness? Let us explore Sonia's case a little further.

Mapuche Medicine and the Social Body

I found Sonia's story puzzling. Why did José's diagnosis of a "great evil" seem so much more attractive than the doctors' diagnosis of "*sistema nerviosa*", when both types of diagnosis were somewhat diffuse and did not really explain the cause of the suffering in this specific case or provide any exact cure? In fact, Sonia had received a "real" diagnosis, that of depression, but she did not consider this very significant, as it did not explain the pain in her chest and nor did the treatment relieve her symptoms. José's success probably turned on the fact that he acknowledged *her experience* of illness, making it legitimate, while the doctors seemed to suggest that her pain was not real, that she was "faking" the pain in her heart. Furthermore, the diagnosis of a "great evil" did not correspond to any fixed disease category, mobilizing Sonia herself, and the women in her social circle (mother, sister, daughter), to establish the signs and symptoms which could reveal the nature of her illness. It was precisely the openness of the diagnosis that created a social space for their creative involvement in the process of identification, turning it into an active social matter.

After consulting the doctor, Sonia returned home feeling ashamed of her state, and afterwards started feeling even worse. This might have been due to the stigma of a psychiatric diagnosis, and the fact that the doctor did not recognize all her symptoms as valid. On the other hand, after visiting José she felt that her suffering had been recognized by another person, while the possibility that it might be caused by something external made a remedy seem much more within reach. Gradually Sonia appeared more and more inclined to believe that the "great evil" was, as her daughter suggested, the result of "black magic", of being bewitched by a Mapuche. In medical dialogue with the women in the family, Sonia started recalling occurrences and signs which confirmed this theory, such as the vision of the dark-skinned boy, the bad cheese and the discovery of the book on witchcraft. Yet this interpretation also made her somewhat uneasy, as it probably meant that someone disliked her enough to want to damage her. Ultimately, however, with José's medicine, this was an illness which had a remedy, which could be fought against. In other words, it objectified her bodily state as a site of human and supernatural action and possibly counteraction, of positive and destructive forces and energies. This helped her rework her own experience to find a framework through which she could cope with her bodily state.

Sonia's story was quite typical of the many patients I followed during my fieldwork, with its fragmented and complex notions of cultural identity, its combination of biomedicine and shamanistic practice, and the underlying experience of feeling marginalized in and by the public health system. It was also representative due to the absence of direct reflections on the political reality of Chile, and the perception of being "equal" with Mapuche neighbours. Indirectly, however, Sonia and her family were commenting on experiences of distrust of and being dehumanized by the public health system. Their experiences pointed to the fallacies of the state in claiming to fulfil the needs of its citizens, in this case looking after their health. Being poor or just being a "normal" Chilean means being excluded from real participation in the project of the nation-state insofar as comprising part of a well-functioning health system. Instead, health is primarily a private matter, not a public one. Nonetheless, Sonia maintained contact with the public health system, thereby navigating between the options and resources that the different types of medicine could offer.

While many patients do make use of the public health service, resolving issues of health is ultimately regarded as falling within the domain of the family. Sonia's story was therefore typical in the sense that it revolved around her family, with the exception of the husband, who was reduced to a shadowy figure. I never met him and the women never referred to him. When I asked directly about his part in the management of her illness, Sonia merely said, in resigned tones, "Well, he just lives in his own world." Instead, it was her mother and her daughter who actively tried to help Sonia to get better; not even the institution of marriage offered her any real comfort or support. But José's medicine served the social function of mobilizing the women in Sonia's social network to combat the illness. This point also corresponds with Magnus Course's findings that there is an "open-endedness" to Mapuche personhood that endows them with a certain centrifugal sociality, a desire to expand relationships with others in an outward direction. In other words, a Mapuche person must create herself through a process of engaging with other social beings (Course 2011: 110, 111; see also Gonzalez Galvez 2012; Crow 2013: 9). We can see that for Sonia—a non-indigenous person living in a Mapuche community—the medical gaze in Mapuche medicine impelled her to engage with social relationships and a collective body of knowledge. Or, in the words of Gonzales, the medical gaze had become part of her "shared world" (Gonzalez Galvez 2015: 153).

MEDICAL CHOICES AS SOCIAL RESOURCES: THE "KNOWN ABOUT" TAKE MATTERS INTO THEIR OWN HANDS

If we return to the original question of the effectiveness of medicine, it may be recalled that Levi-Strauss emphasized that the shamanic cure was effective because it provided a social myth that integrates and gives meaning to bodily symptoms and misfortune (1949). However, as already suggested in Chap. 1, in Levi-Strauss's work the link between individual body and social/collective body is not explored. Sonia's suffering and José's medicine did not only relate to her individual condition, but also to collective experiences, providing Sonia with a variety of resources that were part of a collective social and political reality. The connection with Chile's "roots", with an indigenous world, was considered a moral alternative to the public health system and the Chilean state; furthermore, José's medicine was seen as something human, personal, natural and pure, which served to empower human beings. In other words, it provided a sense of identity and continuity. However, it also offered a framework of action for Sonia to affect her bodily state within her social world. It is precisely by *not* providing a fixed disease category, with signs and symptoms which could only be read by a health practitioner, that it invited the activation of her social relations in the work of identifying signs and symptoms in order to find the cause of illness.

Whereas the disease category of "depression" implies a conception of an inner state of being, with the health practitioner identifying the illness through the patient's reporting of symptoms in a private and individual setting, in Sonia's visit to José the work of identifying the category was externalized and embedded in both the relationship between practitioner and patient, and *also* within the patient's social world. In this way, the notion of biopower and the regimes of knowledge which serve to structure a patient's understanding and social personality were located not only in the relationship between doctor and patient, but also within the social world and the social values which formed part of the patient's everyday life. In consequence, the planting of the patient within an epistemological and ontological understanding which reflected the society's basic ideological premise suddenly became a tool in the hand not only of the practitioner, but also of the social relations surrounding the patient (Taussig 1992).

In this chapter it has been argued that the nature of disease categories is fundamentally different in the two medical traditions. The practice of the biomedical doctor is based on defined, established disease categories, while the patient's subjective experience and the experience of his or her social relations are mostly only relevant in order to identify signs and symptoms that correspond with the categories. Through the establishment of a bio-medical disease category, the patient's symptoms are officially acknowl-edged and recognized within his or her social world, though not always according to the patient's own perception of the nature of the illness. The patient's body thus becomes an isolated identity that is discerned and judged through fixed biomedical categories. This hierarchical relationship between doctor and patient can lead to the conclusion that the patient is not really ill, his or her set of symptoms are not acknowledged as valid—a negative experience increased by the patient's feelings of dissatisfaction with the medical attention provided in the public health setting. On the other hand, in shamanistic practice, while the shaman, as the one who has the knowl-edge to see an illness, might be as much of an authority figure as a biomedi-cal doctor, the use of a disease category which focuses on causality rather than a set of symptoms—that is, the shaman's medical gaze—calls for much broader intersubjective involvement. Therefore, the therapy management group acquires a more crucial role. Being sick in shamanistic practice there-fore links the patient with his or her social environment. Sickness becomes a "collective practice" which involves collective action as well as a search for signs of immoral acts. Hence the biopower, the moral regulation of the human body, is externalized into the social community. Sickness becomes a statement which involves the rest of the community. Consequently, the diagnostic process is embedded in a social process whereby patients negoti-ate personhood and notions of self, in which their relationship to the social environment is a horizontal one characterized by intersubjectivity.

REFERENCES

Agger, I. & S.B. Jensen. 1996. *Trauma y Cura en Situaciones de Terrorismo de Estado. Derechos Humanos y Salud Mental en Chile bajo la Dictadura Militar.* Santiago: Ediciones Chile America CESOC.

Aguirre, S.M., Philippi, L., Artigas, D. & Obach, A. 2003. *Mitos de Chile: Diccionario de seres, magias y encantos.* Sudamericana.

Alonqueo, M. 1979. *Instituciones religiosas del pueblo mapuche: Ngillathún, Ul. uthún, Machithún y Ngeikurrehwen* (Vol. 7). Ediciones Nueva Universidad, Pontificia Universidad Católica de Chile, Vicerrectoria de Comunicaciones.

Bacigalupo, Ana Mariella. 2001. *La Voz del Kultrun en la Modernidad: Tradicion y Cambio en la Terapeutica de Siete Machi Mapuche.* Santiago de Chile: Ediciones Universidad Catolica de Chile.

Bacigalupo, Ana Mariella. 2004. The Mapuche Man Who Became a Woman Shaman. *American Ethnologist* 31: 440–457.

Bacigalupo, Ana Mariella. 2007. *Thunder Shaman. Making History with Mapuche Spirits in Chile and Patagonia*. Texas: University of Texas Press.

Bacigalupo, Ana Mariella. 2016a. *Shamans of the Foye Tree. Gender, Power, and Healing among Chilean Mapuche*. Texas: University of Texas Press.

Bacigalupo, Ana Mariella. 2016b. The Paradox of Disremembering the Dead: Ritual, Memory, and Embodied Historicity in Mapuche Shamanic Personhood. *Anthropology and Humanism* 41.

Bacigalupo, Ana Mariella. 2018. The Mapuche Undead Never Forget: Traumatic Memory and Cosmopolitics in Post-Pinochet Chile. *Anthropology and Humanism* 43(2): 1.

Boccara, Guillaume. 2002. The Mapuche People in Post-Dictatorship Chile. *Ètudes Rurales*. No. 163/164. Terre Territoire Appartenances: 283–303.

Bonelli, C. 2012. Ontological disorders: Nightmares, psychotropic drugs and evil spirits in southern Chile. *Anthropological Theory* 12(4): 407–426.

Bonelli, C. 2014. What Pehuenche blood does: hemic feasting, intersubjective participation, and witchcraft in Southern Chile. *Hau: Journal of Ethnographic Theory* 4(1): 105–127.

Borzutsky, Silvia. 2006. Cooperation or Confrontation between State and the Market: Social Security and Health Policies. In: Silvia Borzutsky & Lois Hecht Oppenheim (eds.), *After Pinochet: The Chilean Road to Democracy and the Market*. Gainesville: University Press of Florida, pp. 142–166.

Caniuqueo, Sergio. 2006. Siglo XX en Gulumapu: De la fragmentación del Wallmapu a la unidad nacional Mapuche. 1880 a 1978. In: Pablo Marimán, Sergio Caniuqueo, José Millalén, Rodrigo level. Eschucha Winka. Cuatro ensayos de Historia Nacional Mapuche y un epílogo sobre el futuro. Satiago, Lom Ediciones, pp. 129–218.

Citarella, Luca, et al. 1995. *Medicinas y Cultura en la Araucanía*. Santiago de Chile: Editorial Sudamericana.

Collier, Simon & William F. Sater. 2004. *A History of Chile, 1808–2002*. Cambridge: Cambridge University Press.

Course, Magnus. 2011. *Becoming Mapuche. Person and Ritual in Indigenous Chile*. Chicago: University of Illinois Press.

Crow, Joanna. 2013. *The Mapuche in modern Chile: a cultural history*. University Press of Florida.

Cruz-Coke, R. 1992. The Expulsion of the Jesuits (1767) and its impact on Chilean medicine in colonial times. *Rev Med Chil* 120(9): 1062–1069.

Dowling, Jorge. 1973. *Religión, Chamanismo y Mitología Mapuches*. Santiago de Chile: Editorial Universitaria.

Eliade, Mircia. 1964. *Shamanism: Archaic Techniques of Ecstacy*. Bollingen series LXVII. Princeton, NJ: Princeton University Press.

Faron, Louis. 1964. *Hawks of the Sun: Mapuche Morality and its Ritual Attributes*. Pittsburgh: University of Pittsburgh Press.

Faron, Louis. 1968. *The Mapuche Indians of Chile*. New York: Holt, Rinehart and Winston.

Faron, Louis. 1969 (1961). *Los Mapuche: Su Estructura Social*. Mexico: Ediciones Especiales.

Foerster, Rolf. 1993. *Introducción a la Religiosidad Mapuche*. Santiago de Chile: Editorial Universitaria.

Foerster, Rolf. 1996. *Jesuitas y Mapuches 1593–1767*. Santiago: Editorial Universitaria.

Foucault, Michel. 1979. *The History of Sexuality. Vol. 1: An Introduction*. London: Penguin Books.

Foucault, Michel. 1994 (1973). *The Birth of the Clinic: An Archaeology of Medical Perception*. New York: Vintage Books.

Giaconi, Juan. 1994. Proyecciones de las reformas introducidos en el sector de salud durante el Gobierno de las Fuerzas Armadas (1973–1990). In: Ernesto Miranda (ed.), *La Salud en Chile. Evolucion y Perspectivas*. Santiago de Chile: Centro de Estudios Publicos, pp. 257–273.

Giminiani, Piergiorgio Di. 2012. *Tierras ancestrales, disputas contemporáneas. Perteninencia y demandas territoriales en la sociedad mapuche rural*. Santiago: Ediciones Universidad Católica de Chile.

Gonzales Galves, Marcelo Ignacio. 2012. Personal Truths, Shared Equivocations. Otherness, Uniqueness, and Social Life among the Mapuche of Southern Chile. PhD in Social Anthropology. The University of Edinburgh.

Gonzales Galves, Marcelo Ignacio. 2015. The truth of experience and its communication: Reflections on Mapuche epistemology. *Anthropological Theory* 15(2): 141–157.

Grebe, María Ester. 1972. La Cosmovisión Mapuche. *Cuadernos de la Realidad Nacional* 14: 46–74.

Hacking, Ian. 1995. *Rewriting the Soul: Multiple Personality and the Sciences of Memory*. Princeton, NJ: Princeton University Press.

Han, Clara. 2012. *Life in Debt. Times of Care and Violence in Neoliberal Chile*. London: University of California Press.

Janzen, John. 1978. *The Quest for Therapy: Medical Pluralism in Lower Zaire*. Berkeley, Los Angeles, and London: University of California Press.

Kirmayer, Lawrence. 1988. Mind and Body as Hidden Values in Biomedicine. In: M. Lock & D.R. Gorden (eds.), *Biomedicine Examined*. Dordrecht: Kluwer Academic Publishers, pp. 57–93.

Kirmayer, Lawrence. 2004. Explaining Medically Unexplained Symptoms. *Canadian Journal of Psychiatry* 49(10): 663–672.

Kleinman, Arthur. 1986. *Social Origins of Distress and Disease: Depression, Neurasthenia, and Pain in Modern China*. New Haven: Yale University Press.

Kuramocho, Yosuke. 1991. *Mitologia Mauche. Colección 500 años*. Quito: Abya-Yala.

Latcham, Ricardo. 1924. *La Organizatión Social y las Creencias Religiopsas de los Antiguos Araucanos*. Santiago de Chile: Imprenta Cervante.

Latcham, Ricardo. 1928. *La Prehistoria Chilena*. Santiago de Chile: Soc. Imp. Y Lit. Universo.

Lévi-Strauss, Claude. 1968. *The Origin of the Table Manners: Introduction to a Science of Mythology*. New York: Basic Books.

Low, Setha. 1994. Embodied Metaphors: Nerves as Lived Experience. In: Thomas Csordas (ed.), *Embodiment and Experience*. Cambridge: Cambridge University Press, pp. 139–162.

Ministerio de Salud, Gobierno de Chile. 1998. *Diagnostico y tratamiento de la depresion en nivel primario de Atencion*. Dept. *programas de las personas*. Unidad de Salud Mental. Serie MINSAL 03- Guias Metodológicas SM no.3.

Ministerio de Salud [Minsal]. 2006. *Avances de la salud en Chile*.

Minsal. Gobierno de Chile, Ministerio de Salud. 2003. *Resultados 1 Encuesta de Salud*.

Minsal. Gobierno de Chile, Ministerio de Salud. 2017. *Encuesta Nacional de Salud 2016–2017*. Primeros resultados.

Miranda, Ernesto (ed.). 1994. *La salud en Chile: Evolucion y perspectivas*. Santiago de Chile: Centro de Estudios Publicos.

Montecino, Sonia. 1999. *Sueño con Menguante: Biografía de una Machi*. Santiago de Chile: Editorial Sudamericana.

Núñez de Pineda, F. 1863. *Cautiverio feliz y razón de las guerras dilatadas de Chile*. Santiago: Imprenta de Ferrocarril (Obra original publicada en 1673).

Organización Panamericana de la Salud. 2002. *La salud pública y la organizacion panamericana de la salud en Chile (1902–2002). Cien años de colaboración*. Santiago de Chile: Organización panamericana de la Salud.

Pinto, Jorge. 1988. *Misioneros en la Araucania 1600–1900*. Temuco: Ediciones Universaidad de la frontera, Serie quinto centenario.

Rosales, Diego. 1989 (1674). *Historia general del reino de Chile*. Valparaiso: Imprenta de El Mercurio.

Saldivia, Sandra, et al. 2004. Use of Mental Health Services in Chile. *Psychiatric Services* 55: 71–76.

Stewart, Carmen López. 2004. Chile Mental Health Country Profile. *International Review of Psychiatry* 16(1–2): 73–82.

Taussig, Michael. 1992. Reification and the Consciousness of the Patient. In: Michael Taussig (ed.), *The Nervous System*. New York and London: Routledge, pp. 83–111.

Torri, Maria Costanza. 2012. Intercultural Health Practices: Towards an Equal Recognition Between Indigenous Medicine and Biomedicine? A case study from Chile. *Health care Anal* 20: 31–49.

CHAPTER 4

Indigenous Disease Categories, Medical Dialogues and Social Positions

With her nice knee-length skirt, pageboy haircut, gold teeth and gold jewellery, Albina signalled the lifestyle of a typically well-off mestizo woman. Her illness story was a theme that she liked to bring up in conversation. She related how she had suffered from an affliction related to the work of evil forces (wekufes) or witches (*brujos*). It began when one day she suddenly collapsed and fell unconscious. Afterwards she did not remember anything about the incident, waking at three in the morning vomiting dramatically without being able to move; later she could only raise herself from the bed with the help of her mother. After the collapse she began having illness attacks, which she describes as susto. These normally started with a sudden loss of the ability to speak, at which point she would try desperately to find someone nearby who could support her, because she knew that she could collapse at any instant. Her family described the expression on her face and in her eyes as "total terror". The attacks came at weekly intervals. She went to a doctor who diagnosed her as suffering from nerves, and she was treated for a while by the "kind" Dr Cordero at the public hospital in individual therapy sessions. Dr Cordero, however, was killed during Augusto Pinochet's military coup in 1973, and Albina did not have the

This is a revised chapter, published as Dorthe Brogård Kristensen (2010). The Shaman or the Doctor? Disease Categories, Medical Discourses and Social Positions. Giovanni Pizza & Helle Johannessen (Eds.). AM: *Rivista della Società italiana di antropologia medica* (SIAM).

103

means to continue to attend private therapy sessions. Instead, she was assigned to Dr Silva, the head of the psychiatric ward in the public hospital. Here the resources for treating the patients were scarce and, according to Albina, mostly consisted in the prescribing of medicine and hospitalization or, as she put it, the offer to commit her to the psychiatric ward to be "locked up with the mad ones". Although she felt that Dr Silva's treatment decreased the frequency of attacks, she was terrified of accusations of being psychologically "bad" or "insane", or of being told that she was imagining things which were not there. At this point, she explained to me, she started treating herself with indigenous medicine, with a completely successful outcome: her attacks stopped.

Since treating her sickness, Sebastian the shaman (machi) had treated her father, mother and son. Her son had been suffering from a mal. Albina related how he had been really well-off, the owner of a house and four cars, when he started to lose his cars one by one; at the same time, he began to feel unwell when in his house, and suffered from insomnia, apathy and constant weeping. He also often saw a man who appeared beside him during the night and heard the sound of strange birds. She explains all this as products of human evil and envy—of wekufes. However, with Sebastian's medicine her son had recovered his health.

In this chapter I address the relationship between illness experiences, disease categories, social class and ethnic relations. During my fieldwork I found that the indigenous diagnosis of susto and mal was very widespread among Mapuche, but also among Chileans, like Albina, defining themselves as mestizo; that is, those with mixed Hispanic and indigenous ancestry.[1] Both types of diagnosis rely on the concept of wekufe or forces of evil (Montecino 1985; Citarella et al. 1995). A person is diagnosed with mal when the cause of symptoms is witchcraft, which has introduced objects into the body of the victims, such as insects/vermin (bichos), reptiles or what is called a "living hair" (*pelo vivo*).[2] Susto means, literally, "fright", and is produced by an encounter with wekufe, which are generally believed to have been sent by a sorcerer. In some cases, susto can also be produced by a traumatic and frightening event.

[1] Out of 30 patients interviewed during my fieldwork, 10 reported symptoms which they identified as susto. Three of these were male and seven female; five of the latter were mestizo women, two were children. All had other diagnoses, mostly depression/nerves, and in two cases they also suspected witchcraft to have been involved. The diagnosis of mal is even more widespread: out of 30 patients, 26 believed or had suspected that witchcraft was involved in their affliction. In this group nine were mestizo women.

[2] These objects enter the body through eating food or beverages bewitched by a sorcerer. The evil force then installs itself inside the victim's body, most commonly in the stomach, sucking the blood and life force.

The symptoms of both include insomnia, bodily swellings, lack of energy and appetite, paleness, vomiting and often visions of the evil forces. The Mapuche view evil as something that attaches itself to people, thereby causing experiences of feeling trapped, weakened, contaminated and confused (Bacigalupo 2007: 75). Birds, insects, cats and dogs are regarded as possible messengers of evil forces, sent by a sorcerer or witch; frequently the destructive force inserts itself into the victim's body, where it starts growing. Many told me that the Mapuche often curse Chileans, causing them misfortune, although it is not uncommon for Chileans to pay the indigenous to send a wekufe. One of these is the *witranalwe*, or cowboy demon, which is described as a man on a horse with a large hat and shining spurs. Created by witches out of femurs recovered from cemeteries, the *witranalwe* often appears at night, blocking the road or path that the person needs to travel (Course 2011: 34). Wekufes are impossible to catch as they often change shape and manifestation, appearing as an animal, a bird, the skin of a sheep which turns out to be alive, or as the crying of a baby or the sound of a bird singing (*twu twu*).

Here I focus on the case of Albina since she, as a mestizo with symptoms of both susto and mal, represented a group of patients that was very salient among those who consulted the Mapuche shamans. The case of Albina is interesting because, although a mestizo, she suffers from symptoms derived from indigenous disease categories which apparently cannot be linked to either a biomedical condition or her self-ascribed ethnicity. The question to be explored is this: If having a Mapuche illness is not connected to a set of organic symptoms, why does Albina then suffer from an indigenous illness?

In this chapter, by analysing Albina's case and comparing it to the cases of two Mapuches[3]—Rosario and Alvaro—I suggest that the value of

---

[3] Susto and mal are, as already described in Chaps. 1 and 3, quite widespread. In order to get an idea of the use and prevalence of different medical practices and explore existing knowledge of Mapuche illness as well as developing a socio-economic profile of patients who suffer from Mapuche illness, I carried out a survey in six different areas in and around Temuco with 120 respondents. The survey was designed with the assistance of a local sociologist and carried out by three local assistants as a simple household survey. According to the findings from the survey, 22% of respondents reported having suffered from susto, and 17% said they had suffered from mal. I was intrigued to see how many mestizo women attended machi medical consultations. The survey supported a negligible gender bias in the spread of susto, as women were only slightly overrepresented. Of the 26 persons who reported that they were suffering from susto, 12 were men and 14 women. That mestizo women apparently dominated in terms of numbers might not be an indication of a higher prevalence of these illnesses and diagnosis among women, but due to the simple fact that women often attend medical consultations on behalf of their family members. Furthermore—

indigenous diagnosis is that it serves as a means for expressing and negotiating a vulnerable position: that of belonging to a downwardly mobile group in a context characterized by modernization and privatization of the health system (Sontag 1991; Crandon-Malamud 1986). To do this I explore experiences of categories such as class and culture, which highlight aspects of olvido, the social forgetting of inequalities in relation to class and ethnicity. I also explore how Mapuche medical dialogues and medical practices become a means to negotiate and establish social bonds between persons who share the same social positioning, in this case Mapuche and the landless and unemployed mestizo. This serves as a counterstrategy to the asymmetrical and hierarchal relationship perceived by the patient to exist between the poor and the biomedical doctor, allowing illness experiences and Mapuche medicine to become resources through which patients navigate and make allies across interethnic boundaries with individuals in a similar social position, despite a perceived difference in ethnicity.

MEDICINE AND POWER RELATIONS

An assumption that is fundamental to my work is that the articulation of illness experiences and medical choices is connected to social and political processes and embedded in political power relations. The practices and politics of the body serve to regulate and control the individual body and the population, but might also be regarded as sites for resistance to the process of standardization, regulation and control (Turner 1992: 10). This resonates with Libbet Crandon-Malamud's point that medicine itself can also be considered as a resource through which people negotiate social positions (Crandon-Malamud 1991: 139), a view founded on the classic anthropological problem of the relationship between body and society, as already described in regard to the notion of the social body. That means that a vision of the body—and in this case, of bodily practices and medical practices—can be regarded as a reflection of social relations and the social world. In this way, a medical diagnosis like susto might represent a symbolic statement of a social position.

A general position within development theory is that modernization destroys, or at least changes, indigenous culture. Yet, as pointed out by several authors, exactly the opposite has been taking place in a number

as I argue in this chapter—it serves as a strategy to position themselves within their social environment and to gain access to health care.

of cultural contexts where the use of indigenous medicine has increased (Koss et al. 2003; Nichter and Lock 2002). Similarly, there is widespread use of indigenous disease categories and medical practice in a section of society in Southern Chile, where indigenous medical practice is both a resource and a means for the articulation of a social order and the establishment of egalitarian social bonds. Through analysis of the cases of Albina and Rosario, I show how common experiences seem to unite their approaches to, and perceptions of, the nature of bodily symptoms as well as the possibility of managing and healing them; this appears through their medical dialogue with neighbours and family as well as the anthropologist.

Some authors have suggested that susto is an idiom for expressing psychosocial distress (Rubel et al. 1984); I, rather, propose that the diagnosis of susto connects the patient with an indigenous medical practice which serves as a means for negotiating ethnic relations and social position within the framework of the state. Here I resort to the theories of Libbet Crandon-Malamud, who argued that medical dialogues (or what people say about their social world through the idiom of medicine) are statements about political and economic realities (Crandon-Malamud 1986: 463). Following Crandon-Malamud, indigenous diagnoses of susto and mal are explored as a window onto the study of social processes and as a way to state and negotiate a position within a socio-political reality. The diagnostic process that takes place in medical dialogue can therefore be considered a social arena, wherein the construction of identity and the negotiation of social and power relations take place. In this way, these dialogues can be regarded as demonstrating the social processes taking place as well as one of the means by which they take place (Crandon-Malamud 1986: 463, 473).

MEDICINE, CULTURE AND SOCIAL CLASS

Since the foundation of the Chilean republic, the mestizo has been considered the ethnic base of Chile, while the indigenous population has been regarded merely as a remnant of the old Chile, who should be subjected to a process of civilization and integration into the modern nation-state. However, as a consequence of state politics, the indigenous and poor mestizo populations share and compete for the same scarce resources, with regard to both land and medicine. Since their "pacification" between 1881 and 1884, the Mapuche have increasingly been integrated into national society, a process accelerated by their continuous loss of territory. With the democratic governments of Eduardo Frei (1994–2000) and Ricardo Lagos (2000–2006), some of the indigenous territories were returned to indigenous owners, but this did not come close to satisfying the needs of the rural Mapuche population. As a result, mestizo farmers and Mapuche have increasingly been forced to co-exist and share the same resources in rural areas (Mallon 2005; Kristensen 1999, 2000). It is also possible to identify a narrative of sameness between the two groups, for instance in the claim that the relationship between Mapuche and non-Mapuche has throughout history been characterized by peaceful, happy co-existence, and that they have mixed to the degree that they share the same land and cultural roots (Richards 2013: 67). It is, however, mostly mestizo landowners who support this version of history, while the Mapuche often refer to social injustices and exploitation as part of their relationship with non-indigenous landowners.

Poor mestizos and Mapuche also share the same medical resources. The official health system today consists of a combination of private and public services (as described in Chap. 3). The proclaimed goal of the creation of this mixed system was to provide the user with the possibility to choose freely between public and private health services, but having a good income allowed the provision of good health insurance and improved the chances of maintaining good health. Thus, "good health" was regulated by the politics of the state through the relationship between income and health insurance. As suggested by Nicolas Rose (2006), state politics based on the idea of individual freedom also paves the way for state control over the medical practices of the population. The health system created in Chile became one that was based on users' access to health insurance. Private insurance became part of this (obligatory) state model for the worker to keep in good health. In reality, the public health system was assigned to the lower social strata in Chile. As described in Chap. 3, it is characterized by insufficient resources, limited services in rural areas, poor and decaying infrastructure, low salaries, lack of medical devices and medicine and long waiting periods (Borzutsky 2006: 150–151). This system has, in some respects, failed to fulfil the expectations and needs of the user, as exemplified by Albina's case. Furthermore, in modern Chile where both indigenous people and Chileans feel alienated and experience conflict and growing economic equalities, accusations of witchcraft are increasing (Bacigalupo 2016: 17).

ALBINA AND ALVARO

The first time I met Albina was in the Mapuche pharmacy when she brought in her Mapuche neighbour whose son, Alvaro, was seriously ill; she also wanted a check-up for her father and herself. In her case it seemed that the reason for visiting the Mapuche pharmacy was to socialize with her neighbours rather than to solve a serious health problem. She talked in a lively way with everyone in the waiting room, commenting on her visits to different shamans, most recently to seek treatment for her father's illness. She had previously visited two shamans, Sebastian and José Caripan, who both diagnosed him as suffering from a condition of "too much liquid around the heart". She regarded it as a proof of the validity of Mapuche medicine that her father had received a similar diagnosis from two practitioners.

Sebastian was very well-known in the urban Mapuche community, especially for the flamboyance of his attire: a colourful headscarf which, on special occasions, was decorated with feathers, a very good-quality poncho and heavy Mapuche jewellery. Sebastian was Catholic, wearing a Christian cross and sometimes referring to himself as a kind of Christ figure due to his healing powers. In addition, he often appeared on television, for instance in the yearly military parade on Independence Day (18 September). Sebastian normally made a diagnosis after looking at the patient's urine, or on the basis of the patient's clothes or identity card. Among his patients he was known as a very powerful shaman.

At the consultation Albina greeted Sebastian cordially, just like an old friend or relative, and commented on his performance and participation in the Independence Day military parade, which had been broadcast on national television. She had brought her father's urine and entered the consultation room with a small plastic bottle containing the sample. When Sebastian made the diagnosis (nervous stomach ulcer, pains in spine, waist and bladder) she seemed more interested in knowing what medicine to take for her migraines. Sebastian advised her to take *pila pila*, a medicinal plant, and told her that she could buy it in the countryside. "No problem," she replied, "I can easily obtain it. I am a very dear friend to my Mapuche acquaintances."

After the consultation, Albina talked about another machi, José Caripan, whom she also knew very well, and commented on his difficulties with the tax authorities as something "which should not happen; the machi ought not to pay tax. Yes, they have even entered his house and caused problems there." Her manner was as self-assured as that of an aficionado of Mapuche culture with intimate, inside information. Her neighbour also knew José Caripan and joined the conversation, revealing that her son was affected by witchcraft (a mal) when he was 15 years old. Now he was 22 and, according to his mother, had a relapse once a year, when he would have a serious panic attack and stop eating and sleeping. At such times they had to perform a ceremony to treat him for this affliction. Albina, due to her concern for the neighbours, had offered to accompany the neighbour to her "favourite" machi, Sebastian.

The boy himself just sat, speechless and apathetic, while Albina and his mother told people in the waiting room about his afflictions and experience of being bewitched. What I found interesting was that Albina, a self-identified mestizo, was professing herself to be an expert on Mapuche culture and explaining where to find treatment for a so-called mal. In doing so, she, like many others I had met who identified themselves as Chilean and mestizo, challenged my original assumption that having a Mapuche illness or a folk illness was connected to articulation of an indigenous cultural identity. Albina did not acknowledge herself as Mapuche, nor pretend to share the Mapuche lifestyle; however, she shared the idiom of indigenous disease categories with knowledge and intensity, and actively showed and expressed her alliance with Mapuche medicine.

Though from different ethnic groups, Alvaro and Albina shared biographical backgrounds; namely, having been placed in the specific community due to political processes. Albina's father, once a poor landless worker, received his plot of land during Pinochet's time, when the contra-agrarian reform after the military coup in 1973 resulted in the transfer of indigenous land to landless mestizo with the aim of producing economic growth. Now the process had been reversed, and Alvaro's parents had received a plot of land from CONADI (National Institution of Indigenous Peoples) that had been bought with governmental funds from a mestizo owner. Thus, Albina and Alvaro's shared rural lifestyle was the result of shifting governmental policies which had placed them in similar social positions. While they identified themselves as belonging to two different ethnic groups, they acted with apparent solidarity in the sharing of the scarce resources in an indigenous community. Alvaro had migrated to Santiago, and Albina's son now lived and worked in Temuco. It was the son who gave Albina the gold jewellery, which created a somewhat false impression of her lifestyle, as her estate was, in fact, quite modest. The jewellery, however, helped her to signal a successful mestizo profile. Albina and Alvaro both commented on the impact that changing governments had had on their lives. Politics as a theme in itself was, however, apparently not of much interest as a topic of conversation; in contrast, the medical dialogue was the idiom through which they articulated their everyday existence.

WHY MAL AND WHY SUSTO?

When Crandon-Malamud enters the discussion of culture-bound syndromes with her study on susto, she does so by switching the question from "what is susto?" to "why susto?" She describes it as a common illness throughout Latin America, with the following symptoms: "restlessness in sleep, listlessness, loss of appetite, weight loss, disinterest in dress and personal hygiene, loss of energy and strength, depression, introversion, paleness, and lethargy"; susto can also lead to "high fever, diarrhoea, and vomiting, occasionally it can lead to paralysis and convulsion" (Crandon-Malamud 1983: 156).

Revising earlier research on susto, she outlines two approaches to the study of "culture-bound syndromes": the first considers such syndromes as psychological/psychosocial, as a culturally appropriate way to express hysterical anxiety (Gillen 1948) or as social role stress within a cultural context (Rubel 1964); the second is based on the assumption that culture-bound syndromes have organic causes, in this case hypoglycaemia (Bolton 1981), which are hidden "in the mists and mires of exotic cultural expression" (Crandon-Malamud 1983: 153). As a starting point, Crandon-Malamud points to the problematic of deciding whether culture-bound syndromes are psychosocial or physiological, as both alternatives fail to acknowledge the significance of the indigenous system of logic. She dismisses the first explanation (social role stress) due to the fact that so many infants apparently suffer from susto: in the area where she worked, susto was reported as the second highest cause of the death of infants under the age of one year. In other words, she finds it unlikely that an infant can die of role stress (Crandon-Malamud 1983: 157). A purely psychological approach, she warns, obviates the assumption that culture, mediated through symbolic systems, plays an active role in the illness process.

Crandon-Malamud also argues against the theory of susto as the exotic manifestation of an authentic medical disease such as hypoglycaemia. This is not to deny the possibility that susto might have physiological causes; on the contrary, she holds that physiological causes in relation to the symptoms of susto might be relevant, not only in connection with hypoglycaemia, but also with a range of other biomedical diagnoses such as gastroenteritis and malnutrition. However, she observes, studies of susto have showed that no single pathology could be identified. This argument is identical with that of an interdisciplinary study published the year after Crandon-Malamud's article, which concluded that patients who were diagnosed with susto could be considered ill from a biomedical point of view, mainly suffering from infective and parasitic diseases or anaemia, yet no single organic syndrome or disturbance was found. The study concluded that susto could not be regarded as a syndrome or be classified as a disease in a medical sense, but rather as a local way of articulating and dealing with social stress. It was, therefore, concluded that many of what are known as culture-bound syndromes are, in fact, not syndromes in the strict medical sense but, rather, local ways of explaining and dealing with illness (Rubel et al. 1984: 87).

Crandon-Malamud further notes that Bolton's (1981) search for organic causes does not explain why people with such a wide range of symptoms and pathologies are diagnosed with the same disease category. If, however, "culture-bound syndromes" (in this case susto) cannot be linked to a biomedical condition, then, she concludes, something else is going on. She proposes that the reason that people choose the diagnosis of susto has to do with negotiation of social inequalities and power relations, due to the fact that "any diagnosis of an illness, perhaps especially *susto*, is a social process that depends on and affects social, economic, political and ethnic relations" (Crandon-Malamud 1983: 154). Consequently, she suggests that rather than focusing on "why certain classes of people are diagnosed with *susto* rather than other classes of people", the focus can be switched to "why certain classes of people are diagnosed as suffering from *susto* rather than from some other illness category" (ibid.). She proposes three levels of analysis in the diagnosis of any illness, especially relevant to susto in this case: What causes the symptoms diagnosed as susto within a given environment? What is its underlying meaning? And, finally, what is the relationship between its meaning and the socio-cultural context, which leads people to diagnose symptoms as susto? In the next section I follow Crandon-Malamud's suggestion and compare the case of Albina with that of a Mapuche woman—Rosario—in order to explore the relationship between illness experience, social class and ethnic identity.

DIFFERENT LIVES, SHARED EXPERIENCES

Albina and Rosario are in many ways at a similar life stage and share, to a large extent, the same socio-economic reality. They are both in their late 50s, have grown-up children who have moved to a larger city, and they have both lived in rural as well as urban areas. Both live a very modest life, surviving as itinerant vendors of home-produced products, in their cases cheese and flowers. The financial support of their children helps them to make ends meet. Although without any formal education, they both appear to be strong, independent and articulate women, who managed to break out of violent marriages to alcoholic men.

Another common feature is their perception and use of the Chilean health system. Both make use of biomedicine in case of illness, and ensure that they and those close to them do not miss any medical check-ups. Rosario suffers from high blood pressure and rheumatism, Albina from varicose veins. The consequences of distancing themselves from the bio-medical system would be fatal, they claim; they would thereby risk being denied treatment in an emergency, as well as the opportunity to get a medi-cal certificate in case of illness or death. Dying in the house of one of the "clandestine" practitioners, the *machis, meicas* and *yerbeteras* (herbalists), puts both the practitioner and his or her family at risk of difficulties such as a law suit. They do, however, accept the diagnoses they get from the medi-cal doctors, and also take the medicine they have been given, even though this is often not considered "good medicine" (*buena medicina*), usually due to what they consider an inadequate diagnosis. The doctor's medicine might alleviate the physical symptoms, but it neither accepts nor explains the complex combination of symptoms—physical, psychological, social and often also spiritual—which the patient experiences.

In other words, the loyalty of the women does not lie with the Chilean doctors and their medicine; far from it. Indeed, the following phrase was often repeated: "I really do not trust doctors." This distrust contrasts with their almost blind confidence in Mapuche medicine; of course, not in all of the practitioners of Mapuche medicine, but in the healing practices themselves, when they are well practised. Who is a good practitioner, who has treated whom for what and on which occasion, and what was the cause of the illness—these are themes that are constantly discussed. As with most other patients I met, they had their "favourite" practitioner of Mapuche medicine, who was sought on those occasions when the biomedical doc-tors could not provide a satisfactory diagnosis. The relationship with this practitioner was one spanning generations, and also included the illness stories of several family members and neighbours; in this way one could almost say that the practitioners of Mapuche medicine were granted the status of family doctor. Everyday conversations often concerned illness stories; in these medial dialogues, trust and mistrust in social relations were expressed through the identification with good and constructive or evil and destructive forces. In other words, spiritual forces and witchcraft were a crucial part of the social reality of these women, particularly expressed through the fear of witches (*brujos*) who used evil forces—the wekufe—as their intermediaries. The experience of having been influenced by wekufes was one that both women revealed in their talk of illness stories and medical choices.

"*POR ESO TENGO FE*"—THE REASON WHY I HAVE FAITH

Both Albina and Rosario can be considered what could be called "medical resource persons". Their way of making a social entrée is characterized by illness stories incorporating tales of successful healing by a Mapuche practitioner. They make use of their experiences and knowledge of medicine, especially Mapuche medicine, as a social resource; they enjoy conveying their medical knowledge and their own illness experiences and are often consulted in situations of illness; they also most happily volunteer to accompany relatives and neighbours to their "favourite" medical practitioner. Due to the many years of consulting machis, they have gained a solid knowledge of Mapuche medicine and medicinal plants, so they are often asked for medical advice, and they grow those medicinal plants that are considered an important source for maintaining good health in their gardens.

Hardly surprisingly, I met them when they were accompanying a patient: Albina was with a young Mapuche neighbour and Rosario was with her sister-in-law, Nancy, a 50-year-old mestizo woman. Through medical dialogue between mestizo and Mapuche, they both reflected on the nature of illness, mostly on whether the patient was affected by a natural or spiritual illness and the social implications. Thus, medicine served as a symbol of a social position that also provided an idiom through which they expressed values, evaluated social relationships and explored different options for action (Crandon-Malamud 1991: 151). Both Albina and Rosario consulted their favourite practitioner due to "spiritual" suffering, what some would call a "Mapuche illness"; that is, they suffered from an illness with both physical and psychological symptoms, which did not fit a biomedical diagnosis, especially in relation to pain, which had no organic explanation.

Rosario had suffered for 14 years from an affliction which did not have a biomedical explanation. Her stomach became enormously swollen, even though her only nourishment was soup; at the same time, she suffered from what she described as an intense "pain in the bones", in her knees and legs but also at her waist, in her head and especially in the intestines, which felt as though they were falling out or as if something was moving around inside them. She felt totally drained and exhausted and also suffered from insomnia. Furthermore, she described an extreme paleness produced by "the lack of blood". At home strange occurrences started to happen—the house started creaking, although it was totally new, and she constantly had the feeling of being haunted by something, but when she turned around nothing could be seen. She went to a doctor who diagnosed her as suffering from swellings which might be the beginning of rheumatism. On a later occasion he diagnosed her as suffering from a cold, with high blood pressure, and he gave her aspirin and vitamins. As the doctor did not prescribe medicine that could give her relief from her symptoms of exhaustion and swelling, Albina began to search for another diagnosis and treatment.

During my fieldwork I often heard stories similar to this, of all types of illnesses which doctors often dismiss as problems with the nervous system, anxiety or depression, or simply treat with aspirin. Among patients in Southern Chile, when illness occurs which cannot be treated with biomedicine or herbs, there is always a lurking fear that it has been produced by a spirit or a human witch, who has used spiritual powers to produce misfortune and sickness. To the practitioners of indigenous medicine, sickness is considered a sign of imbalance and is often diagnosed as an affliction produced by external forces, spiritual as well as human, that have made a pact with evil forces, the so-called wekufe. While patients consult Mapuche practitioners for many different types of illnesses—among them a number of so-called natural illnesses—supernatural/spiritual illnesses (*males*) or Mapuche illnesses (*mapuche kutran*) like *kalku kutran, infitun, trafentun, perrimonton* or susto are the most common reasons. These illnesses are thought to be caused by an unbalance or conflict between the patient and his or her social environment and/or transgression of a social norm. Health practices—including practices for bewitching or preventing and counteracting witchcraft—are often used to explain the patient's trust and preference for Mapuche practitioners. The signs that are used to identify a witch are often articulated and shared.

MEDICAL PRACTICES, SOCIAL POSITION
AND CULTURAL IDENTITY

The belief in, and concern for, practices of health and illness, among them practices for preventing witchcraft (*contras*), are facets of everyday life that Rosario and Albina share as a fundamental part of their reality. Rosario told me how she had been diagnosed as having an insect (bicho) or a living hair inside her, feeding on her. This was a product of witchcraft. Or, in other words, she suffered from a mal, the popular or mestizo term for *kalkutun*, an illness caused by witches (*kalkus, brujos*) through *infitun*, or poison given in drink or food. This diagnosis was first made by a herbalist; Rosario did not, however, follow the treatment. Later she heard rumours about a famous shaman and went to José Caripan, who made the same diagnosis and succeeded in treating and curing her. Albina is sure that she was poisoned with a glass of red wine. Consequently, in their articulation of illness the women move in a similar universe with similar diagnoses, where external forces are considered the actors when other more natural factors fail to provide any explanation.

In other ways, however, Albina and Rosario differ in their life situations. While Rosario has remarried and now lives an urban life with her new husband, Albina continues her rural life, sharing a house with her parents. What is even more interesting is that Rosario identifies herself as pure "Mapuche", and Albina as "mestizo" or "Chilean". This did not, however, seem to make much difference to their medical choices, though some differences could be traced in the role that medicine plays in their self-identification. In this chapter I argue that this is due to the fact that disease categories—especially indigenous types of diagnosis—represent a possibility for the articulation and management of certain social experiences which the women share. By discussing their symptoms in medical dialogue within their social relations, they draw on disease categories that shape their self-perception and identification.

Applying Crandon-Malamud's approach, the fact that Albina is mestizo becomes especially interesting. In her own research she too had wondered why so many mestizo adults in Bolivia suffer from an indigenous disease which is mainly thought to affect indigenous people. In the case of this present study, one could pose a similar question: Why do mestizo women suffer from diseases which are framed with an indigenous logic and labelled "Mapuche illnesses", which explain sickness as soul loss; that is, as a product of fright, spirit attack (susto, *trafentun*) or as witchcraft (mal, *kalku kutrun, infitun*)? Why does the medical dialogue of Rosario, Albina and Alvaro's mother, contain similar statements claiming that certain afflictions are inherently spiritual? During my fieldwork it became clear that it is quite common for people who identify themselves as mestizo to accuse Mapuche culture of being "backward", yet ally themselves with Mapuche culture and indigenous cosmology when it comes to medical choices. This was especially salient—as explored below—in the case of mestizo Chileans who refer to themselves as "marginal", "poor" and/or "exploited". This highlights Crandon-Malamud's suggestion that biomedicine cannot accommodate the psychological needs of the downwardly mobile, the "victims" of "modernization" (Crandon-Malamud 2003: 28). To these people, who perceive themselves as marginalized and even "betrayed" by the Chilean health-care system, Western biomedical care seems to offer no solution. Consequently, when Alvaro, Rosario and Albina share a medical choice, they are making a statement about their social reality on several levels. Similarly, why people choose a certain disease category could, as Crandon-Malamud proposed, be answered on different levels.

Firstly, by sharing their experiences of susto and mal, the women are making a statement about their social relationship and their use of indigenous medicine as a means of establishing and strengthening social bonds. In other words, choosing an indigenous disease, a spiritual rather than Western aetiology, has different social and ethnic implications. While Albina tried to project herself as a well-off mestizo city dweller, her lifestyle was in fact much more modest and characterized by a daily struggle to make the most of scarce resources. Establishing egalitarian social bonds with her Mapuche neighbours was a logical strategy in order to constitute herself within her present reality in an indigenous community. Through the use of indigenous medicine, she adopted aspects of indigenous identity. The diagnosis of susto and mal linked the women together in a shared idiom of being possible victims of external forces, an idiom of social vulnerability and "loss" of control. In other words, the use of indigenous medicine and diagnosis produced resonance between life experiences, feelings of vulnerability and their current social environments. Moreover, the women preferred Mapuche medicine due to the horizontal relationship between practitioner and patient that made it possible to establish bonds of solidarity with both the practitioner and his group of patients. The result is that, despite ethnically identifying with two different cultural categories (mestizo and Mapuche), the women share a similar social position. Secondly, the use of a Mapuche disease category points to the inefficiency of biomedicine and thereby implies a distancing from official ways of explaining and treating illness. By sharing their symptoms in medical dialogue rather than in "confessions" to their medical doctors, the women partially negotiate the asymmetrical power relations between doctor and patient.

An interesting question is whether Albina's apparent downward mobility (in the direction of her poor indigenous neighbours) does in fact lead to improved health care (Crandon-Malamud 1986: 472). In her own viewpoint that was definitely the case, as she shared Rosario's perception that Mapuche medicine was the only available medical alternative for health care. Rosario phrased it in the following way:

> So many people have died. The people do not know how to get medicine, they have no places to go, then the sickness gets worse and then that is just the end. But at least—thank God—thanks to don José [her machi] I have recovered to last a couple more years.

While I have emphasized the connection between susto and mal and a vulnerable social position, it is important to stress that ethnicity does play a role in diagnosis. That is, vulnerability was associated with being indigenous. In contrast, being Chilean white was associated with a more secure and impregnable position. Thus, Rosario commented:

> Do you know what, miss? The Chilean people are much stronger than the Mapuche; if a Mapuche knows about this [witchcraft practices] and uses it against a Chilean it will not be as effective as if a Chilean person performs witchcraft against a Mapuche. The Mapuche are much more vulnerable.

In other words, vulnerability is connected to being poor, but also to being indigenous. However, in the case of the indigenous, this vulnerability is also connected to practices to counteract destructive, evil forces; that is, indigenous practitioners are considered experts on witchcraft, as "knowers of the secrets of nature", which is why Albina stressed the importance of maintaining good relations with her Mapuche neighbours:

> I tell you, we have never been racist; we have never discriminated against the Mapuche. We are completely surrounded by Mapuche, and I hope that one day they will look upon us as kind people. We feel equal with the Mapuche; we have never looked down upon these people. And they are so good to us when they perform their rituals; we don't even have time to go to all the places where they invite us.

This makes it clear that sharing medical practices was not associated with shared ethnicity; rather, Albina constantly opposed herself ethnically to her Mapuche neighbours. However, through shared experiences of social position, Mapuche medicine became a resource, both as a symbol for a socially vulnerable situation as well as a resource to create social bonds and to gain access to health services.

MEDICAL PRACTICES AND SOCIAL CLASS: UNFULFILLED DREAMS OF MODERNITY

In her work, Crandon-Malamud proposed that medical dialogues are statements of social and political reality; however, her focus is primarily on inter-ethnic relations rather than an analysis of class relations (Crandon-Malamud 1983, 1986). In contrast, in my material, the diagnosis of susto and mal appears to be connected with articulation and negotiation of a social position and of class relations. Focusing on the nature of the social experiences that seem to unite Mapuche and mestizo patients in their use of medicine and in the medical dialogue, in what follows I compare Albina's susto to other cases of susto and mal in order to analyse why mestizo women so often appear among the patients of the Mapuche shamans.

In his article "Susto: An Illness of the Poor" (1998), Avis Mysik suggests that susto is closely connected to class relations, observing that its victims are primarily poor peasants and landless labourers, the working poor and the downwardly mobile. Mysik stresses, however, that this conclusion does not challenge the hypothesis that susto involves some combination of psychological, physiological and social factors, merely pointing out that little research has addressed the relationship between susto and class position. Mysik regards susto as a symbolic statement of an individual's position in the community, whether self- or other-perceived. In addition, he argues that the symbolic statement made by mestizos falling prey to the malady is one of downward mobility. By comparing Albina's case to other instances of susto and mal, it is possible to identify the themes that might unite the sufferers as a group. Albina, as a mestizo woman with susto and mal, was quite typical of many patients I met. It is interesting, therefore, to explore the link between an indigenous diagnosis and social positions, values and class relations.

Generally, Mapuche medicine is characterized by its users as the medicine of the "modest people" (*gente humilde*). A 40-year-old landless mestizo woman observed, "The majority of the rich people go to the doctor;

that might be the reason that they tell us that they cannot give us medicine, because we cannot afford to buy it." A woman who worked with her husband as a shoemaker also suffered from susto and depression; she explained to me that as an urban modern citizen she had felt "obliged" to go to a doctor. This was part of the package offered by the government, providing access to education and health for the workers. The shoemaker analysed the situation in the following way:

> After the introduction of the public health system the population grew so much that the medicine they offered became insufficient, and now when they offer medicine they just greet you and then tell you to leave. No, for the poor they do not offer good medicine.

Another mestizo woman working at a market selling fruit and vegetables said:

> It ought to be more complete, but the fact is that medicine today is too expensive. An operation costs you so much; just to have a medical examination costs you so much, I believe that many people just die because they cannot afford a biomedical examination; in the end what is left to us is the natural medicine [Mapuche medicine]. So many people are just left to die because they cannot afford to have an operation. I believe that the government is responsible for this, because they do not provide for and take care of the poor people. So many people are left without work, and then they cannot afford health insurance and so they cannot provide health for the family. In the end the family suffers, because there is no greater pain to a mother than to have a sick child and not be able to solve the problem. I know this from my own experience.

This woman's statement, similar to those of many others, indicates that, after the introduction of neo-liberal politics, the prospects of gaining guarantees for health and education were limited to one section of society while others were completely left out. The shoemaker complained of having her dreams of getting an education and a good life destroyed due to her very limited income. Now she sees her life as quite hopeless:

> How awful is this life of mine. But that is how it is. Perhaps I did choose this life myself; there is a saying that each person chooses his life. Perhaps I did choose it myself, but I did not choose this situation; I wanted to progress in life, I wanted my family to progress, I wanted many people to progress together with me, but that did not become a reality.

In these statements the effect of the privatization of social security becomes clear. Firstly, a division was created between social strata in their access to medicine; and secondly, the entire life situation became a private matter, to be solved, if at all, by the core family. If an expectation is not fulfilled, it is the individual who is regarded as responsible. This corresponds to Pinochet's neo-liberal model, with its emphasis on personal freedom. The flip side of this vision is the experience of social isolation and a lack of confidence in the social authorities; namely, biomedical doctors and priests. This particular woman told me very private details of her life—as did many other patients I interviewed—meanwhile claiming that she hardly ever confessed her inner thoughts. Many other women had similar comments. Although identifying herself as Catholic, one woman said about Catholic absolution, "I simply don't like to go there to confess." Another said, "You cannot tell the doctor what you think might be causing your sickness, nor report all your symptoms, as they do not believe the same things as us." Yet another advised me never to tell personal things to a medical doctor because "they might use it against you afterwards". As mentioned in Chap. 3, one woman even said about the medical doctors, "If you don't leave a cheque of guarantee to pay for the medical treatment, they just let you die at the entrance [to the building, without letting you in]." To this remark a man commented, "The doctors have made a huge business of our bodies." Compounding the problem, due to the lack of social security the consequences of being sick were, in many cases, almost disastrous. One woman described how medical neglect in an operation to remove her husband's appendix had left him unable to work for a year, leaving the family to survive on savings and charity. Today she treats her own susto, a condition which she thinks is caused by her desperate social situation, through the machi, Sebastian.

Hardly surprisingly, my work as a medical anthropologist collecting illness stories was easy. The interviews were shaped as a medical dialogue, which constituted the statement of their social situation by these women; they also represented a strategy and a social resource. When choosing to tell their illness stories in medical dialogues with peers rather than to medical doctors, the women were negotiating their social position by avoiding entry into the hierarchical relationship with the authorities. In this way the medical dialogue becomes a way to creatively negotiate power relations by establishing social bonds. Furthermore, medicine became a strategy for action that obviated the need to adopt a political strategy; in their individual versions of the reasons for their unfulfilled dreams of a good life, no political action was imagined. A landless mestizo woman and her husband had dreamt of becoming owners of a small plot of land; now they only had a shelter provided by their patron in return for services such as looking after livestock. I asked if the situation would change if a socialist president was elected and they responded, "If only it would change, but that would be like trying to get a star down from heaven." They even claimed that it might get worse with a socialist president, as the effects might include fewer industries and, therefore, less work. In a similar vein another woman said, "We just stick to our work, to what we can do; I do not understand much of politics, not much; I only vote because I am supposed to vote, but I am not really into politics." A taxi driver said, "No matter who is elected, we just have to work like hell."

All these people—both self-identified Mapuche and mestizo—shared experiences of social and economic marginalization that could be described as "downwardly mobile", in which the good life of Chilean citizens, including access to work, health and education, was not fulfilled. This observation apparently confirms the hypothesis that susto and mal are expressions of role stress and a product of psychological and social stress. However, my argument, which I develop in the following chapters, is that Mapuche diagnosis and medical practice form a valid alternative to bio-medicine because they also provide a sense of agency—that is, social values that help the downwardly mobile cope with their situation—offering a strategy for dealing with a challenging social situation.

"The forces of evil always go after the most fragile, the most weak," many people told me. Therefore, lack of work and of good health was regarded as a circumstance that increased the possibility that a person might be affected by wekufes. In the same breath, the comment was also an explanation of misfortune, with its emphasis on how human greed and envy often result in witchcraft. Many of the women I met reported that the search for medicine makes them feel better, or even that they feel better just by being on their way to meet the Mapuche practitioner, or on arrival, before being given any medicine at all. A mestizo woman described the effect of indigenous medicine "as having been in foggy mist, and then you just see everything clearly again". Another said that on her way to her machi (don José) she already felt better:

> His medicine makes me feel good. It helped counter the susto I had, though of course it [the susto] still hits me but not as [much as] in that time when I felt really so bad, that I did not feel like me, when I lost the affection for

my home, for everything. It feels as though when I am leaving to go there [to don José] I already begin to feel better; I arrive and it is as though things just become calmer.

CONCLUSION: MAPUCHE MEDICINE AS A MEANS TO EXPRESS, EXPLAIN AND COPE

In this chapter it has been shown that indigenous cosmology provides a means of experiencing and acting in relation to a trying social situation, firstly through the establishment of social bonds, secondly by creating a space for action in the negotiation of power relations. Albina's case is an example of how indigenous medical practice facilitates the establishing of social bonds; as a medical resource person, Albina is constantly in contact with her favourite health practitioners, which makes her feel well.

As demonstrated, Rosario and Albina, although from different ethnic backgrounds, share many common experiences and a common social arena. For both of them, Mapuche medicine provided social bonds and medical knowledge which worked to counteract the influence that evil forces have on human lives, and both used the idiom of wekufes in connection with experiences of loss of life force and energy, associated with destruction and death. However, the latter belief also has its counteraction, as both women use the Christian cross to ward off evil as well as attending the healing rituals of their favourite machi. The principal element the two women had in common was their social position. They share and negotiate the same resources—land, work and medicine—with access to biomedical care considered especially scarce. In a context of privatization and modernization, their relationship to official medicine and medical doctors was characterized by a feelings of marginalization and lack of influence. Thus the women shared a vulnerable social position, which they negotiated in medical dialogue. The use of indigenous medicine became a symbol of a social position that supplied a resource for negotiating social and power relations. Through medical dialogue they established egalitarian bonds and expressed social values; being "indigenous" was associated with vulnerability and loss of control and became a means to express a socially difficult situation. Furthermore, indigenous medical practice involved a negotiation of power relations and an explanation for sickness and misfortune through a vision of the duality of good and destructive forces.

REFERENCES

Bacigalupo, Ana Mariella. 2007. *Thunder Shaman. Making History with Mapuche Spirits in Chile and Patagonia*. Texas: University of Texas Press.

Bacigalupo, Ana Mariella. 2016. *Shamans of the Foye Tree. Gender, Power, and Healing among Chilean Mapuche*. Texas: University of Texas Press.

Bolton, R. 1981. Susto, Hostility, and Hypoglycemia. *Ethnology* 19: 261–276.

Borzutsky, Silvia. 2006. Cooperation or Confrontation between State and the Market: Social Security and Health Policies. In: Silvia Borzutsky & Lois Hecht Oppenheim (eds.), *After Pinochet: The Chilean Road to Democracy and the Market*. Gainesville: University Press of Florida, pp. 142–166.

Citarella, Luca, et al. 1995. *Medicinas y Cultura en la Araucanía*. Santiago de Chile: Editorial Sudamericana.

Course, Magnus. 2011. *Becoming Mapuche. Person and Ritual in Indigenous Chile*. Chicago: University of Illinois Press.

Crandon-Malamud, Libbet. 1983. Why Susto. *Ethnology. An International Journal of Cultural and Social Anthropology* XXII: 153–169.

Crandon-Malamud, Libbet. 1986. Medical Dialogue and the Political Economy of Medical Pluralism: a Case from Rural Highland Bolivia. *American Ethnologist* 13(3): 463–477.

Crandon-Malamud, Libbet. 1991. *From the Fat of our Souls: Social Change, Political Process, and Medical Pluralism in Bolivia*. Berkeley: University of California Press.

Crandon-Malamud, Libbet. 2003. Changing Times and Changing Symptoms: the Effects of Modernization of Mestizo Medicine in Rural Bolivia (the Case of Two Mestizo Sisters). In: Joan D. Koss-Chioino, Thomas Leatherman & Christine Greenway (eds.), *Medical Pluralism in the Andes*. Psychology Press, pp. 27–42.

Gillen, J. 1948. Magical Fright. *Psychiatry* 11(4): 387–400.

Koss, Chionino, Leatherman T. & Christine Greenway (eds.). 2003. *Medical Pluralism in the Andes*. Psychology Press.

Kristensen, Dorthe Brogård. 1999. Chile. In: *The Indigenous World 1998–1999*. København: Iwgia, pp. 121–124.

Kristensen, Dorthe Brogård. 2000. Chile. In: *The Indigenous World 1999–2000*. København: Iwgia, pp. 142–148.

Mallon, F.E. 2005. *Courage tastes of blood: The Mapuche community of Nicolás Ailío and the Chilean state, 1906–2001*. Duke University Press.

Montecino, Sonia. 1985. *Mujeres Mapuche: El Saber Tradicional de la Curación de Enfermedades Communes*. Santiago de Chile: CEM.

Mysik, Avis. 1998. Susto: An Illness of the Poor. *Dialectical Anthropology* 23: 187–202.

Nichter, Mark & Margaret Lock (eds.). 2002. Introduction: from Documenting Medical Pluralism to Critical Interpretations of Globalized Health Knowledge,

Policies and Practices. In: Mark Nichter & Margaret Lock (eds.), *New Horizons in Medical Anthropology*, pp. 1–35.

Richards, P. 2013. *Race and the Chilean miracle: Neoliberalism, democracy, and indigenous rights*. University of Pittsburgh Press.

Rose, Nicolas. 2006. Governing "Advanced" Liberal Democracies. In: Aradhana Sharma & Akhil Gupta (eds.), *The Anthropology of the State*. Malden and Oxford: Blackwell Publishing.

Rubel, A. 1964. The Epidemiology of a Folk Illness: Susto in Hispanic America. *Ethnology* 3: 268–283.

Rubel, Arthur, O'Nell Carl & Rolando Collado-Ardón. 1984. *Susto: A Folk Illness*. Berkeley and Los Angeles: University of California Press.

Sontag, Susan. 1991. *Illness as Metaphor: Aids and its Metaphors*. London: Penguin Books.

Turner, Brian. 1992. *Regulating Bodies: Essays in Medical Sociology*. London and New York: Routledge.

CHAPTER 5

Being Mapuche in Modern Chile: Illness Experiences, Medical Choices and Social Positions

Life is hard. It is like a growing forest; at a distance it looks so pretty and has such a nice smell, but if you start looking more closely, you see that some trees are drying out. Little by little, the small trees suffer because there are other huge trees that do not permit the small ones to grow. It's really true, nature is so cruel.

This is how Leonardo, a young Mapuche man, presented his vision of everyday life in contemporary Chile. Young, single, unemployed, without any formal education and with a serious drinking problem, his future prospects indeed seemed rather poor. Furthermore, he was struggling with an illness problem which began when he was working in the city as a machine operator; he tells of how he felt so apprehensive during that time that he had attacks of nerves. Suddenly he would become frightened for no apparent reason, yet the fear was often so intense that he became dizzy and had stomach pains and visual disturbances. "After eating I got these attacks. I just felt awful, the whole day became just awful." He also described a feeling of being incapable of changing his life, which produced a state of utter despair, so overpowering that he felt like he was "choking".

Leonardo went to see a medical doctor, who told him that he apparently had no "real" disease; rather, his health problems were caused by "too much drinking" and "nerves". The doctor subsequently diagnosed him as suffering from depression and nerves and prescribed anti-depressants, but his condition did not greatly improve and he eventually stopped taking the medicine. Leonardo's grandmother suggested that he might have been

© The Author(s) 2019
D. B. Kristensen, *Patients, Doctors and Healers*,
https://doi.org/10.1007/978-3-319-97031-8_5

bewitched and made him a medicine (*contra*) against witchcraft or spirit attack. This made him vomit, and afterwards he felt some relief but did not recover completely, so his search went on. He consulted an indigenous practitioner who diagnosed him as suffering from "a problem with the spirits", or *wenu kutran*, and gave him an antidote to the harmful influence of spirit attack.

I met Leonardo at the urban centre of diagnosis and treatment (El Centro Medico) connected with the Mapuche pharmacy in Temuco, when he had been ill for about a year; he complained of having spent all his money on medicine, most of it on being examined for ulcers and on medicine for depression. He had heard about the herbalist Maria, a 55-year-old rural woman working at El Centro Medico, and decided to consult her. Maria, introduced at the beginning of Chap. 1, worked as a herbalist, calling herself a *lawentuchefe*. She was an evangelical Christian and often used Christian orations as part of her treatments. Maria did not identify herself as Mapuche by blood but, an orphan, she was raised by Mapuche parents and said she felt truly Mapuche. She wore typical Mapuche clothes when at work, but dressed mestizo fashion (blouse and skirt) in her daily life. Maria claimed to have received the gift of healing through dreams that have made her able to "feel" the patients' health problems by putting her hand around their wrists and feeling their pulse. Maria had knowledge of medicinal plants used to treat many types of afflictions; she often had dreams in which medicines were "shown" to her. She specialized in treating infants, as well as the common complaints of stress and nerves, seeing around 10 to 20 patients a day during office hours (from 10 a.m. to 2 p.m.).

By touching Leonardo's pulse, Maria diagnosed him as suffering from depression, insomnia and pasmo—also called *aire*—the so-called natural illness (*re kutran*) that is produced by a sudden change in the environment. The symptoms of pasmo are—as in Leonardo's case—headaches and sometimes eczema. Maria explained that Leonardo had an inner heat which had no outlet. She calmed him, telling him that his condition was not very serious and that he would soon feel better. She sold him some drops from the Mapuche pharmacy and a bottle of her own home-prepared medicine. After this treatment he felt much better and calmer, particularly, he explained to me, in a moral sense.

In the previous chapter I suggested that mestizo patients' use of Mapuche medicine was linked to their negotiation of class relations and cultural identity. In this chapter I also focus on the relationship between illness experiences, medical choices and categories of class and culture, but through the experiences of another group of patients who were likewise well represented in the medical consultation of Mapuche practitioners: young Mapuche with a history of migration for work. I explore the illnesses and social situation of Leonardo and Alvaro, two young Mapuche men, and their stories of migration and social change, which typify the experiences of the younger generation of Mapuche born in the countryside whom I met in medical consultations.[1] Having neither land nor jobs, they both left rural life to work in the city, but due to their illnesses they returned to the countryside, only journeying to the city in search of a medical cure. It is important to note that these two men chose practitioners in an urban setting and not a more traditional rural one.

Why do actors perceive a certain medicine as being effective? Looking for answers to this question, I examine the use of symbols in illness experiences, the potential to articulate connected processes and the relationship between medical practitioner and patient. The theoretical aim is to understand the links between the illness experience and socio-political reality, the latter, in this case, being the context of modernization and social change that is so much a part of the neo-liberal model (see Chap. 2). My perspective is inspired by theories of embodiment that consider the body not only as imbued with social meaning, but also as a historically situated and active force for expressing and negotiating a socio-economic and political context (Lock 1993: 142). In this chapter I consider the links between individual bodies/bodily symptoms and socio-political processes. However, rather than focusing primarily on the cause of the illness in order to explain the bodily symptoms as a sign, metaphor or representation of a situation characterized by oppression and distress, I examine why a disease category makes sense in a particular social situation, what possibilities it provides for agency and the social implications of choosing a particular disease category and treatment. Thus, the use of medicine is regarded as a resource in the constitution of agency and complex identities.

In her book *Life in Debt: Times of Care and Violence in Neoliberal Chile* (2012), Clara Han introduces the term "neoliberal depression"—characterized by bodily pains, racing thoughts and sleepless nights (2012: 129)—which she describes as produced by the social inequalities of the neo-liberal system: in other words, as representative of the olvido of modern, capital-

---

[1] A study from 1992 revealed that eight out of ten Mapuche live in the city, in densely populated areas (Pérez 2000).

ist-state-produced social inequality. Expanding on this theme, in this chapter I argue that medicine is increasingly effective according to the degree to which it resolves a "referential dissonance" between a personal life story and socio-political reality. The latter term is inspired by Han's (2004) article on what she calls the "traumatic present of late capitalist Chile", where she defines referential dissonance as a gap that emerges between the historical languages that inform subjectivities (2004: 169). When a patient perceives a medicine to be effective, it will be argued that a referential resonance has occurred between medical practitioner and patient: I define this as a match between an individual's personal experience and social environment and the practitioner and his or her medical practice. This relationship allows the patient to be projected forwards (Das and Kleinman 2001: 22); that is, it allows the patient to enter a framework for action that is consistent with both his or her life experiences as well as the moral and social world of which she or he forms a part.

EMBODIED METAPHORS IN ILLNESS EXPERIENCE AND MEDICAL PRACTICE

In classic theories of medical anthropology, the focus in the analysis of illness experiences is on the metaphors people use to describe their sufferings (Kirmayer 1988; Scheper-Hughes and Lock 1987; Lock and Scheper-Hughes 1990; Low 1994). The use of metaphors to describe a condition has been regarded as "strategic" (Low 1994) and as a way for the body to express itself and act in a social situation. In the same vein, sickness is regarded as "not just an isolated event or unfortunate brush with nature" (Lock and Scheper-Hughes 1990), but rather as a "cultural performance" involving "the embodied person living out and creatively responding to their assigned place in the social order" (Scheper-Hughes 1994: 235).

"Nerves" or nervios is a typical example cited in the literature of an embodied metaphor for social distress (Coker 2004), which has been treated as a culture-bound or culturally interpreted syndrome (Guarnaccia 1993). In clinical literature, "nerves" has been referred to as "somatization" and as a state of pathology, an "unconscious generally maladaptive amplification and exaggeration of psychological symptoms by the individual sufferer" (Scheper-Hughes 1994: 234). In anthropological works on "nerves" inspired by theories of embodiment, it has been suggested that it would be more useful to move away from the body/mind dualism and the interpretation of "nerves" as a product of psychosocial distress to its analysis in its social and political context. Thus the affliction has been linked to structural inequalities in society and has been analysed as a socially sanctioned vehicle for the expression of bodily distress (Lock 1993). Nancy Scheper-Hughes's analysis of nervios among shantytown dwellers in northeast Brazil exemplifies how an illness manifestation may be regarded as a metaphor for the expression and negotiation of a social situation (1993). In her work, the idiom of nerves is considered a metaphor for hunger and malnutrition, one that has been adopted due to the dangers of openly discussing the causes underlying these problems. The pitfall of this approach, however, as has been pointed out by DiGiacomo (1992), is that it focuses very much on the body as a locus for resistance, "that it recruits suffering into the service of an ideological agenda", thereby neglecting the biological and random aspect of illness episodes and reducing them to a form of protest (DiGiacomo 1992: 126).

The aim of the following analysis, inspired by recent work on embodiment, is to move away from considering idioms of distress primarily as pathological expressions and metaphors for social and psychological distress. Rather than focusing specifically on the metaphor inherent in bodily complaints, the aim is to place the articulation of illness within a context of medical pluralism and, through this, to explore how medical choices of diagnosis and treatment are tools for articulating and negotiating a position within a social, cultural and political reality. Instead of analysing illness as resistance and a metaphor for social distress, I will see how illness experiences offer opportunities for both a symbolic statement of a complex social situation which unifies the significance and experience of the alienation and fragmentation of social ties, and also the reworking and possible transformation of that situation.

Being Mapuche in Modern Chile

As already described in Chap. 2, the Mapuche played a crucial part as the heroes of liberty in the war against the Spanish colonizers. However, in modern Chile, Mapuche culture is not considered part of the national culture and Mapuche social and economic marginalization has increased over the last few decades. This development has today divided the Mapuche population into two segments. One comprises a poor rural population, which survives on small plots of land with economic assistance from family members who have migrated to the city. Culturally, the rural Mapuche population is considered to be relatively autonomous, as they still maintain some Mapuche traditions such as the practice of the fertility ritual *nguilla-tun*, and some also preserve the original language, Mapudungun. However, in many areas, due to the strong influence of evangelical Christianity, many Mapuche traditions have been replaced by the practice of Christian ceremonies, while the younger generations often distance themselves from traditional medicine and rituals (Torri 2012: 42; Bacigalupo 2007: 224; Mallon 2005: 235). The other segment of the Mapuche population, the large majority, live in the cities (in Santiago alone they number around 500,000) where they have mixed with the mestizo population. Socially, they are considered one of the lower strata, employed in low-paid unskilled jobs, mainly domestic service and construction.

Officially Chile is recognized as culturally homogenous, and has only recently ratified international instruments for the political recognition of ethnic minorities.[2] As described in Chap. 2, since the 1990s a political Mapuche movement has pursued its goals through the symbolic occupation (*toma*) of estates on the basis of the original documents of indigenous ownership (Títulos de Merced), which were initially granted to all indigenous land.[3] The movement also uses other means of expression such as burning the timber and lorries belonging to logging companies.[4] These conflicts have led to serious confrontations between members of the movement and the Chilean police force, which has prosecuted hundreds of activists through the anti-terror law (Instituto de Estudios Indigenas 2003; Kristensen 1999, 2000, 2001). The conflict between private logging companies, the Chilean state and the Mapuche movement reflects the current ambivalence in Chilean identity politics, as it establishes the image that being indigenous means being left outside the modern state. The indigenous population is, on the one hand, considered to provide Chile with its true and authentic roots and heroic blood; however, on the other, its people are culturally, socially and politically marginalized in the modern project of the nation-state. Chilean historians Gabrial Salazar and Julio Pinto cite the example of

[2] This is founded in ILO Convention 169 from 1988, "Convention concerning indigenous and tribal populations in independent countries".

[3] The Mapuche movement is in fact not a single and united movement, but consists of a number of indigenous organizations, among which El Consejo de todas las Tierras and La Cordinadora have played the most prominent part.

[4] Another conflict between the Mapuche and the state broke out at the Bío Bío River, where the Spanish electricity company ENDESA planned to construct a series of dams for hydroelectric power.

a university textbook (see excerpt below), which serves to illustrate the prevailing view of the indigenous people in contemporary Chilean society based on the discrimination and racism that I explore in this chapter:

> The Chilean people are still too indigenous; they need to mix with European blood to a greater degree, which will be an initiative to practice economy, reliability and honesty ... It is a requisite to increase immigration in order to improve the race, increase production and consumption levels and raise the human level of our race. (Cited in Salazar and Pinto 1999: 140, my translation)

In a similar vein, a Swiss settler by the name of Luchsinger, who had been in confrontation with Mapuche due to the usurpation of 1200 hectares of land granted to the Mapuche through land titles, declared the following in an interview with the newspaper *Que pasa* (Bacigalupo 2016: 185):

> It is not possible [to give the Mapuche back their land). It would be absolute misery because Mapuches don't work their land. Have you seen the land that the state has bought for them through CONADI? Nothing is left. Not even one tree is standing. They produce nothing. The Mapuche is a predator. He lives from what nature gives him. He has no intellectual capacity, no will, no infrastructure. He has nothing. (*Que pasa* June 18, 2005)

When discussing the cases of the two young Mapuche migrants— Alvaro and Leonardo—I focus on their negotiation of disease categories and cultural identity, as I regard these as a window onto social processes that include unequal power relations and different sets of cultural values: those attached to modern city life as a Chilean wage labourer and the spiritual "Mapuche" values of a rural land-based life. The gap in the historical languages and values that inform their lives is reflected in their medical choices. Here I compare the different possible strategies for articulation and negotiation provided to the patient by the biomedical category of depression on the one hand, versus indigenous disease categories on the other, and the social implications involved in accepting a particular illness category and resultant treatment. The illness stories in this chapter differ from those of the women in the preceding chapter due to their lack of order and coherence. To readers these cases will probably appear both complex and confusing. This is, I suggest, because the accounts reveal gaps in the different historical discourses that informed and influenced the personal life stories of the subjects. To begin with, there is a conflict between the promised comforts of life as a worker in a neo-liberal model, with access to health and consumption, and the reality. Their actual experience as indigenous migrants did not fit this dream, as they both suffered from a fragmentation of social ties and bodily distress and eventually had to give up their jobs and leave the city. Yet the prospect of going to the city to make money and become a "modern" consumer still seems more attractive than the life their families continue to live as poor indigenous farmers, stigmatized, to some extent, as backward and marginalized. This is probably the cause of their ambivalence about their own identities as Mapuche.

This ambivalence was also reflected in the disease categories and bodily metaphors the men used to articulate their illness stories. They used the disease category of depression, an illness—whether seen as biological or psychological—that is regarded as located inside an individual body, the treatment of which, therefore, also focuses on the individual body. This biomedical version has been popularized in Chile, and in Latin America more generally, in the disease categories of "nerves" and the "nervous system" (Low 1994) which, in most cultural contexts, refer to a notion of feeling "out of control". Moreover, an indigenous idiom of distress is implicated in the diagnosis of *trafentun* (susto), *perrimonton* and *kalkutun* (mal). In these categories, disease is regarded as being caused by interference from outside spiritual forces, most commonly depicted as wekufe, the Mapuche word for negative energy; this might be an entity sent by a witch (*kalku*) or an evil spirit working on its own. Due to strong Christian influences in the Mapuche communities (as described in Chap. 2), today a wekufe is often referred to as "mal", "diablo" or "el demonio", all denoting the Christian notion of the devil (Citarella et al. 1995: 336; Foerster 1993). Finally, there is the indigenous disease category of *kastigo kutran*, an illness that is the result of a moral transgression.

LEONARDO

When I first met Leonardo, he thought that his problem was related to pasmo or depression and nerves—as noted above, the folk idiom for "being out of control" which is often used in connection with anxiety; he related this to his excessive playing of violent computer games. Thus, he initially seemed to adopt a disease category that regarded illness as located in the individual body, making it seem manageable, something which could be treated with a medical substance. The nerves might be interpreted as a typical example of an idiom of distress. Unemployed, without financial means and with a heavy alcohol intake, his situation really seemed to be characterized by social and psychological distress, manifested in somatic complaints, a viewpoint which was shared by his doctor as they agreed on the disease category of nerves. Apparently Leonardo did not reflect on the social order that had placed him in this rather marginal social position as unemployed, uneducated and indigenous, although his vision of the life of the forest seemed like a very pessimistic picture of neo-liberal capitalist society. By using the diagnosis of depression, Leonardo envisioned his disease as a private, psychological and individual occurrence which could be controlled through the intake of prescribed biomedicine. In adopting this disease category, he negotiated between dominant and alternative models of reality. By seeing himself as depressed and suffering from nerves, he accepted both a biomedical model of illness and a more popular Chilean version, thereby avoiding the stigma of an indigenous identity, of an inherently superstitious and magical or, in other words, non-modern worldview.

I visited him in the countryside in a rural community or *comunidad* after he had seen the herbalist Maria. Here he presented me with another piece of the illness story, one in which he increasingly seemed to adopt a more spiritual explanation connected to social and moral values quite different from those of "rational" biomedicine, which helped to explain why he considered Maria's medicine effective. I was received by his grandparents and aunts, who served a local Mapuche dish of boiled wheat, *mote*, with Coke, boiled eggs and *sopapillas* (warm fried bread). His parents had left to work in Santiago, the capital, and Leonardo had decided to stay near his grandfather's house in the country. Leonardo's grandfather noted how in the old days so many people died of *trastorno mental*, of madness; at that time there were no hospitals and only the machis knew how to deal with madness, adding that today there were no machis in the area. The influence of the Christian church had here, as in many other areas in the south of Chile,[5] resulted in the disappearance of machis as well as the prohibition of alcohol consumption, participation in games and the practice of traditional Mapuche rituals in the communities, as these were thought to be "demonic" (Citarella et al. 1995: 325). The grandfather also related how many people had been killed during the time of Pinochet and just thrown into the river. One of the murderers was a local policeman, who was still on duty and regularly visited the community.

[5] The number of Pentecostal Christians among the Mapuche has been estimated at 20% (see Foerster 1993). For the role of Pentecostalism in Chile, see Lindhardt (2012).

Although identifying himself as Mapuche, Leonardo did not show any interest in sharing these memories of the destiny of the Mapuche during the military regime. This ambivalence and complex navigation of his position within the social order were underlined in other parts of his story. Though his manner was distant, and he seemed reluctant to engage in conversation about the past, Leonardo happily shared his interest in big towns and city life, as well as memories of his time in high school and in the army. He told how he suffered terribly from the racism of a German teacher, who always referred to the Mapuche as some sort of inferior race. In his time in the army in the south, most of his companions were Mapuche. They had to march for days,[6] living only on beans and mouldy bread; after this he started to drink heavily. He showed me around the plot and told me more about how his affliction started with intense stomach pains when he was working with "that machine". He explained this affliction as depression, which he described as a disease that "does not permit you to be happy, but just stay seated on a chair; even with a comfortable life, this disease will always accompany you. I have this disease and I will always have it." When asked about the cause of his condition, he related it to too much playing of computer games with satanic content in which, for instance, the Christian cross was ridiculed. After this his attacks of susto or fright began, along with his nightmares:

> Once I dreamt that I was in the city wearing a nice suit, and I saw a huge building, and I went to the elevator and expected to ascend, but instead the elevator descended; it felt like being hit, and it just descended and descended. While still in the dream I remembered an elevator accident, where the people were squashed completely, and I thought to myself that I preferred dying immediately than ending up like these people. But I just went down and down and finally hit the ground, then I realized I was in a big hole and everything was dark, and I thought, now I am dead and have ended up in hell. But suddenly I saw this little thing that entered the door, a thing with horns. I did not manage to see the face, but it was so like the devil when it appears in the papers, with a three-pronged fork at its side. And it was laughing and laughing. And then I woke up and felt so bad for days, I felt like I had seen death itself.

---

[6] During my fieldwork, the military practice of long marches was a theme of discussion, especially after a regiment of soldiers had been subjected to a long march in the Andes and had been surprised by a snowstorm during which 47 soldiers froze to death. As most of the soldiers were poor and Mapuche, this was seen by some of the relatives of the deceased as exemplifying the discipline to which the lower classes are subjected as Chilean citizens.

He also ascribed his illness to his amoral behaviour, designating it as a punishment for not living according to a moral worldview. In this way he reproduced the indigenous disease category of *kastigo kutran*, which results from moral transgression and is thought to be influenced by Christianity, being very close to the Christian notion of "sin". He had committed a "sin" by playing anti-Christ computer games, an explanation that made the devil's appearing in his dream seem like an articulation of the loss of values and personal identity, a cruel disfiguration of human relations. He himself described his condition as "being completely lost".

He was also plagued by the presence of spirits. Together with his brother he was working in a storehouse one day when everything started to move. He said: "It was such a strong movement, then a light appeared and we heard footsteps on the roof. We were completely terrified. My father told us that this place was haunted." Following this, Leonardo heard footsteps on the roof over his room at three o'clock each night for two months. One night, his fright intensified by feeling a strong wind and hearing a voice, he woke his brother and they went to his father, who suggested that the steps he heard could be associated with the entity of the wekufe, also referred to as the devil. Often the appearance of a spirit indicates illness related to the supernatural, a notion which Leonardo's symptoms did indeed seem to support. Leonardo also thought that they might be a product of his amoral behaviour, as already mentioned. In such a case a machi would often be considered the most appropriate healer to approach due to their power to expel evil. Leonardo, however, refused to perform a shamanistic ritual of exorcism with the machis, a rejection that reflected the historical reality of strong evangelism in his community. As an aspect of this evangelism, which is very influential in some rural areas, churches have proscribed involvement with traditional practices, especially Mapuche rituals, although elements of the culture have been preserved, including the knowledge and use of medicinal plants.

Instead, Leonardo consulted Maria, the evangelical herbalist, who represented both Mapuche culture and evangelical values. He also began to attend an evangelical church nearby. This apparently helped his condition to improve; he felt much more optimistic and believed that the power of God defended him against destructive, evil influences. Furthermore, he felt good being among other young people who shared his vision of life.

ALVARO

It is interesting to compare the stories of Leonardo and Alvaro, as the two men, although from different rural areas, had similar social positions: in their early 20s, they lacked education and had worked temporarily in the city. Both first presented themselves to me as suffering from "depression" and were treated by a Mapuche practitioner in an urban area. They differed in some central respects, however, as Leonardo lived in a rural area influenced by evangelical churches, while Alvaro's family originated from one with Catholic influences, where they still maintained ritual traditional Mapuche practices. In fact, his mother Elna was the daughter of the local *lonko*, a chief who acts as ritual leader in the performance of the fertility ritual *nguillatun*.

As recounted in the previous chapter, I also met Alvaro at El Centro Medico, together with his mother and his mestizo neighbour Albina. Having lost his job as assistant in a bakery, and due to his illness problems, he had returned from his life as a migrant worker in Santiago. He missed the "fun" of living in the city, but complained about how difficult it was to survive there, economically and socially; furthermore, he suffered from symptoms such as fright (susto), insomnia, headaches, lack of energy, anxiety and the feeling of being choked, as well as from spirit visions and nightmares. Thus, his articulation of his illness, apart from having headaches rather than stomach aches, was quite similar to Leonardo's. Alvaro had decided to consult Sebastian, the machi, rather than Maria. Since the age of 15, Alvaro had often had illness episodes similar to the current one, but had always recovered for a period of time. He had been advised to consult a psychologist, but had refused. His decision to come to Sebastian's consultation was apparently due Sebastian's reputation as a "powerful" machi, who had treated several family members—an aunt and a sister— with good results.

When I met Alvaro, he was isolated and apparently alienated from the world around him; he just sat apathetically, smoking cigarettes, and did not sleep, eat or talk. It was difficult, however, to identify what came first, his illness or his apparent disengagement, although his story seemed to suggest the latter. His neighbour Albina and his mother Elna ascribed his condition to witchcraft practices, but Alvaro himself did not agree; neither did the practitioner Sebastian, who diagnosed him as suffering from "depression" due to an unhappy love affair with a young mestizo girl whom he had met while working in the city. Alvaro confirmed this diagnosis by admitting that his depression was caused by worrying about his love who was, according to him, currently confined in a psychiatric ward because of "madness".

I met Alvaro again after he had been staying at Sebastian's house for a week to treat his depression. He appeared much livelier and instantly started talking about his "health problems". Before her "madness", his girlfriend and he had twice visited a machi, who diagnosed her as suffering from witchcraft and advised her to have a ritual of exorcism (*machitun*) performed. However, her father was evangelical and refused to permit it; according to Alvaro, he had locked his daughter up in the house, where she became very ill. This incident had caused her "madness" as well as Alvaro's own "depression" due to worry.

This diagnosis, however, could not be confirmed, by either doctors or psychologists, as Alvaro refused to see them in the belief that they "only make you suffer more". He had trust only in the Mapuche practitioners, in the machi. His family supported this line of argument by talking in horrified tones of the treatment in the psychiatric wards, of how they just give people pills and subject them to frequent electric shock treatments, thereby reproducing a common vision in Chile of the horrors of psychiatric treatment, described in Chap. 3.

I visited Alvaro a month after his treatment, when he and his family told me more about his affliction while cooking empanados for their guest. The atmosphere was cosy and relaxed, quite a contrast to the topic of conversation—illness and suffering. Alvaro claimed to be a lot better and did indeed seem more articulate, lively and present. He vividly described how Sebastian had treated him for his "depression" by cleansing his brain, which was performed by inhaling a very bitter medicine through the nose. Sebastian had also performed a ritual in front of his *rewe*, his sacred alter. It seemed as though the healing session had provided Alvaro with, or activated, an idiom for his bodily state. Alvaro might be depressed, as Sebastian had diagnosed; however, if this were the case, he expressed his depression through a vocabulary quite distinct from that of biomedicine. Although the diagnosis of susto was not mentioned, Alvaro recounted symptoms which could be associated with it, repeating the word *asustado* (frightened). As mentioned earlier, susto occurs when the soul—the vital force—has been captured by spirits or when a part of the soul has been lost due to a startling or frightening event. The healing procedure consists in the shaman's identifying the incident that led to the loss of the patient's soul, whereupon the shaman's soul travels to rescue the missing part, to wrest it from the negative entity that has captured it and bring it back to the patient. This sometimes happens when talking with the patient in order to identify the incident that led to the soul loss, but this is not always necessary and the shaman may simply carry out the work of healing, giving the patient the medicine that is necessary in order to return the soul and restore the bodily balance.

Another diagnosis, *perrimonton* or "influenced by a spirit vision", also came up when Alvaro offered a brief glimpse of his nightly sufferings: "You see something attacking you, like what you see after death; you feel as though the hour of death has arrived or that you will do harm to yourself, even kill yourself." The energy which haunted him presented itself as a voice talking, which, he claimed, indicated a spirit similar to the one who gave Sebastian his healing power. A shaman is believed to receive his power from a spirit or a vision (*perrimonton*), which is a spiritual call (*llama-miento*). It is a strong energy which, if handled well, could lead to spiritual power; if not approached in the correct way, however, it could lead to destruction. According to Sebastian, this energy was a heritage from Alvaro's ancestor, a powerful energy that had now produced his illness. Here the idiom of shamanistic healing had ways to treat this energy through a set of "body politics", such as the performing of rituals in combination with interaction with the spiritual force that produced the illness.

Alvaro, however, seemed very uneasy about the possibility that he had a "shamanic illness". While it explained his symptoms and gave him a framework for dealing with them, it also implied the adoption of innumerable rules and disciplines that shamans are supposed to follow, an idea which appeared to disturb him: "You cannot marry if you accept this heritage, and if it [the energy force] is not treated well, you can die from it," he commented. "This thing imposes a lot of instructions about how and with whom to live." In order to help Alvaro deal with the energy, Sebastian had advised his patient to forget about his love, to continue his treatment, to leave his parents' house and to return to his urban life. His parents did not oppose this suggestion, but repeated that we should all join the *nguil-latun* ritual in his mother's community of origin the following month. "It is so important to keep in contact with traditions, with our past," his mother Elna said, before telling a story about a mountain that had opened up during one such ceremony. Inside the mountain, the *lonkos* (chiefs) appeared along with two young maidens (*kalfumalen*) who were seated on chairs of gold and silver. Elna spoke about the magic of Indian mythology, which fascinated the anthropologist in me but not Alvaro, who seemed more interested in going to Santiago to earn money, meet girls and have a good time. "The countryside is so boring," Alvaro complained, when he accompanied me to the house of their neighbour Albina, who was waiting with freshly made bread. Of course, they commented when I said goodbye and left their house, their dear Albina was also invited to participate in the ritual.

THE EFFECTIVENESS OF MEDICINE: DISSONANCE AND RESONANCE

Against the background of the two cases just presented, I return to my initial question: What is the relationship between diagnosis, medical choice and social position among the Mapuche in Chile? This is linked to the question of why certain actors perceive a certain medicine to be effective. Here I suggest that the answer to this question can only be reached through an understanding of the link between illness experiences, treatment and social position. Furthermore, I highlight the importance of referential dissonance or resonance between life experience, social environment and medical practitioner.

As already stated, I regard medicines as material objects imbued with social meanings, here focusing in more detail on the symbols in illness experiences and medical practice in order to explore why actors perceive a particular medical practice to be effective. This is important for showing the link between the illness experience, life situation and treatment. In Leonardo and Alvaro's stories, a wekufe, or the devil, represents a symbol in dreams and in medical practice which unifies experiences of alienation and the fragmentation of social ties in the context of the neo-liberal state. The devil or wekufe opens the way for the symbolic work of navigating between opposing social forces, on the one hand positive and on the other destructive. In these cases I found a lack of a direct reflection on the social, moral and political world of the two young men, although their illness experiences draw on elements from the social reality of which they form part. Analysed in context and in relation to social processes, the navigation between disease categories reveals a gap between the languages that constitute the lives of the men. Through the relationship with a medical practitioner, however, the men are able, to some extent, to transcend this gap, which results in an increased perception of the medicine as effective.

In the case of Leonardo's illness experience, the concept of evil, depicted as a wekufe or the devil, was very prominent. According to Bacigalupo, for the Mapuche the devil is associated with savagery and immorality; the capitalistic mentality also contrasts with Mapuche morality and sociality (2016: 61). In a similar vein, Michael Taussig argues that devil belief is a response to what people see as "an evil and destructive way of ordering economic life" (1980: 17). He also explores the notion that devil beliefs are "collective manifestations of a way of life losing its life ... intricate manifestations that are permeated with historical meanings and that register in the symbols of that history, what it means to lose control over the means of production and be controlled by them" (ibid.). He suggests that in a historical context where one mode of production and life is being supplanted by another, the devil is a dramatic representation of the process of alienation; in support of this thesis, Leonardo's illness did indeed start during a period of social change when his agrarian lifestyle was replaced with that of a wage labourer.

Maria's treatment became a compromise between the opposing social forces and languages that informed Leonardo's life. The referential dissonance between the values of the dominant Chilean society and his experience as a Mapuche on the margins of society was mediated through Maria; as a Mapuche healer, she was in opposition to the dominant values but, working in an urban clinic and recognizing and utilizing the diagnosis of depression, she did not fit the non-modern, uncivilized, backward stereotype either. As a result, Leonardo's depression emerged as quite different from the dominant biomedical profile, since he connected its cause to moral and social values which reflected the influence of both Christian symbols and indigenous, spiritual forces. In other words, indigenous disease categories as well as social and moral values underlay the diagnosis of depression. In that sense, Leonardo's vision of his illness and recovery was closely tied to moral values, and his depression did not, in the end, correspond to any biomedical notion of disease, but rather to a perception of illness in which the individual body is affected by spiritual forces and moral acts. Maria's diagnosis seemed to provide a link and a referential resonance with this, operating as she did within Mapuche disease categories which resonated with Leonardo's own perception of illness. What seems peculiar, however, is that both the medical doctor and Maria provided a diagnosis of, and medicine for, depression, but Maria's medicine was apparently more effective. This is, I suggest, due to a referential resonance between

Maria as an evangelical herbalist, the diagnosis provided, Leonardo's life story as a migrant worker and the social environment to which he belonged. One can conclude that his depression was strongly linked to moral values, to the struggle between good and evil forces.

As with Leonardo, Alvaro's case did not have an unequivocal resolution or coherent narrative pattern either. His illness story could be seen as an embodiment of social conflicts and different historical languages. On the one hand, he adopted a "spiritual" worldview, relating illness to the actions of other people (his girlfriend's affliction). He also accepted the diagnosis that he had a shamanistic call (*perrimonton*). However, in many ways he preferred the opportunities provided by modern life in the city, finding them more attractive than the options offered by the medical practitioner, Sebastian, which would involve sacrificing what he thought of as the "fun" of life; rather, he would have to act as the "spirits" told him to. This left him in limbo: his affliction was not completely cured but he felt he was getting better. Thus, Sebastian's diagnosis of depression and his advice to go to the city to get rid of the negative energy served as a compromise which helped Alvaro recover. Sebastian's treatment proved effective because Sebastian embodied and mediated the gaps between languages and the social conflict present in Alvaro's life.

In this case, the referential resonance between Alvaro's illness experience and Sebastian's diagnosis was almost complete; that is, Sebastian's medical practice serve to mediate the gaps that Alvaro experienced between the values of the dominant society, his life as a migrant and his social environment in a rural setting, because Sebastian's diagnosis was consistent with Alvaro's personal experience: Alvaro had already identified a cause which Sebastian confirmed. What seemed to be crucial was the relationship with a practitioner who validated his experience. This apparently brought him back to the social world or, rather, activated one that already existed but was dormant; it also provided a diagnosis and an idiom of suffering, which had a positive impact on his management of the situation. Furthermore, the medical treatment of a machi resonated within the social world of which Alvaro was a part. The argument here, explored further in the following chapters, is that the effectiveness of indigenous medicine (as with other medical practice) lies to a great extent in already-existing social processes and their referential resonance with the diagnostic process, and in the interaction between a personal story, a current social environment and a medical practice.

THE SOCIAL IMPLICATIONS OF MEDICAL CHOICES

Being ill is before all an alienation from the world. (Buytendijk in Leder 1990: 80)

The patient is never totally cut off from the intersubjective world, never totally ill. (Merleau-Ponty 2002: 191)

According to Michael Taussig, the relationship between doctor and patient is more than a technical one, because the social interaction between practitioners and patients reinforces a culture's basic premises in a powerful way. The sick person is plunged into a maelstrom of existential questions concerning life and death. Although the everyday routine of social life is disrupted through the intersubjective relationship with a medical practitioner, the practitioner is given an entry into the psyche of the patient and the possibility of restructuring the patient's relationship to the social world. In other words, the function of the relationship between doctor and patient is to bring the patient back to society and to ground him or her within an epistemological and ontological regime of knowledge that is, ultimately, healing (Taussig 1992: 87). As Susan Sontag (1991) has pointed out, the signs and symptoms of the disease have a material quality but, much more than this, they are also social facts embedded in power relations. The practitioner sees the manifestation of disease as symbols, which he interprets with an eye trained to perceive reality in a certain way (Taussig 1992: 87). The patient's understanding of the world is disrupted through illness, but he or she then acquires, through diagnosis and medical treatment, the possibility of restructuring his or her understanding of the social world.

In his book *The Absent Body*, Drew Leder proposes that illness implies an alienation or withdrawal from the world. Further, he characterizes illness as a disruption of intentional links and, if it involves a stay in hospital (or some other such recovery setting), a spatio-temporal constriction (1990: 80). When the body stops functioning normally, it influences participation in everyday activities, which leads patients to adopt a different kind of gaze: away from the social world and inward, in self-absorption. However, I propose that being ill also implies a gaze *into* the social world, because an idiom for expressing illness symptoms contains the possibility of reintegration into the social world through diagnosis, treatment and articulation. A quest for medicine is therefore closely linked to sociality, becoming a way for the patient to restructure his or her experience in resonance with a diagnosis and a practitioner. In the interaction between practitioner and patient, common cultural and social understandings of the world are highlighted and reproduced. Thus, diagnosis and treatment not only serve to articulate psychological and social distress, but also to provide the individual with symbols and guidelines for action which help to develop a framework for the negotiation of social processes.

Both men initially presented their illness as "depression", thereby adopting a dominant model for their illness. In the biomedical diagnosis, the cause of disease is located within the individual body, and the physical symptoms are regarded as the expression of psychological and social distress. The medical treatment consists of taking biomedicine prescribed by the physician. This illness model implies not only a mind/body dualism (symptoms are seen as not "real", just pathological manifestations of distress), but also a split between a person and his or her environment. The disease is perceived as individual, located within an individual body and requiring the individual body to be healed. By also integrating a "spiritual" diagnosis such as those provided by Maria and Sebastian, the body was presented as an open entity, which could be influenced by external forces, destructive or positive.

Maria's diagnosis of Leonardo established, as has been described, a referential resonance with his life world by combining biomedical notions of depression, the idiom of "nerves" and Christian morality. This became a tool for action by incorporating a dualism between good and evil forces and acts considered as both the cause of, and the cure for, his "depression". By attributing his illness to moral values rather than Mapuche spirits, he was able to avoid the realm of the machis, with its specific rules and disciplines, thereby maintaining a distance from what could be considered a traditional Mapuche worldview. Conversely, in the biomedical treatment for his depression, Leonardo was not given any direct insight into the "soul", only medicines that he had to take to make him feel better; that is, no solution was provided for the referential dissonance between the values of the dominant society and his life experience as a migrant worker. Yet, as Maria suggested, the focus on good forces gave him a certain relief and encouraged him to enter a Christian community. This treatment is not a story of success, but nor is it the opposite; instead, it reflects the power of agency in the constitution of a complex identity.

In contrast, Alvaro's case was a story of successful medical efficacy, which had certain social implications. Alvaro already seemed much better even before he went to Sebastian's house for treatment. It seems as though he had just been waiting for a chance to communicate his version of his afflictions, and here his mestizo neighbour, Albina, provided the social bond that made it possible. Consequently, the meaning was not provided by the diagnosis, it was already present before the diagnostic process; however, through Sebastian's diagnosis he found a framework for coping with his affliction. Alvaro had already actively defined an approach to the management of his affliction which had certain social implications. He had diagnosed himself as suffering from "depression", although the symptoms he described were very similar to those of persons suffering from susto, indicating the work of supernatural forces and reflecting the social world. One can conclude that different diagnoses lead to different implications for what a human being is and for the nature of the relationship between the individual and the social world. In Alvaro's case, his bodily symptoms integrated different types of worlds and therefore different types of diagnosis.

CONCLUSION: MEDICINE, AGENCY AND COMPLEX IDENTITIES

In this chapter I have presented the illness stories of two young Mapuche migrants. Their stories appear to be complex, confusing and fragmentary; this is, I suggest, because they reproduce a gap in the languages that inform their lives, a gap reflected in their use of disease categories and treatments that present a certain cultural confusion and fragmentation. Both men initially labelled their illness as "depression", a model of illness with wide acceptance in society. In the diagnosis of depression, the cause of disease is located within the individual body, and the physical symptoms are regarded as the expression of psychological and social distress. The medical treatment consists of taking biomedicine prescribed by a medical doctor. This illness model implies not only a mind/body dualism in which symptoms are not "real", just pathological manifestations of distress, but also a split between a person and his or her environment.

Leonardo received biomedical treatment for his depression, and in accordance with this model no insight into the "soul" was provided. The fact that Maria also diagnosed him as suffering from depression and gave him medicine, but was apparently more successful in alleviating his symptoms, is possibly due to a referential resonance between Maria as an evangelical herbalist, the diagnosis provided, Leonardo's life story and the social environment in which he participated. Thus his depression was strongly linked to moral values reflecting good and evil forces. In Alvaro's case, the depression was *only* treated by a Mapuche practitioner; this led to the adoption of a disease category wherein the depression was attributed to the working of spiritual forces, thereby establishing a referential link between Sebastian's medical practice, Alvaro's personal experience and his social environment. Furthermore, Sebastian provided a framework for dealing with his situation and linking it to moral values. Hence his treatment was perceived as quite successful.

I have suggested that the medical treatment provided by Maria and Sebastian both embodied and mediated opposing social forces and languages and, through this, provided a framework for action by linking the patient to symbols and social and moral values. The illness experiences of the young men—although operating within the category of depression—escaped being subsumed by the dominant model for perceiving the illness, which locates it within the individual body. In line with the argument presented in this chapter, therefore, their medical treatment could be regarded as creating a referential resonance between personal experience, selfhood, current social environment and medical practitioner which connected them to a moral and social "home"; that is, to a locus for identity and agency. Their illness stories reveal the body as a social and cultural battlefield in the micro-physics of lived experience.

REFERENCES

Bacigalupo, Ana Mariella. 2007. *Thunder Shaman. Making History with Mapuche Spirits in Chile and Patagonia.* Texas: University of Texas Press.

Bacigalupo, Ana Mariella. 2016. *Shamans of the Foye Tree. Gender, Power, and Healing among Chilean Mapuche.* Texas: University of Texas Press.

Citarella, Luca, et al. 1995. *Medicinas y Cultura en la Araucanía.* Santiago de Chile: Editorial Sudamericana.

Coker, Elizabeth Marie. 2004. "Travelling Pains": Embodied Metaphors of Suffering among Southern Sudanese Refugees in Cairo. *Culture, Medicine and Psychiatry* 28: 15–39.

Das, Veena & Arthur Kleinman. 2001. Introduction. In: Veena Das, Arthur Kleinman, Margaret Lock, Mamphela Ramphele & Pamela Reynolds (eds.), *Remaking a World: Violence, Social Suffering and Recovery.* Berkeley, Los Angeles, London: University of California Press, pp. 1–31.

Digiacomo, Susan. 1992. Metaphor as Illness: Postmodern Dilemmas in the Representation of Body, Mind and Disorder. *Medical Anthropology* 14: 109–137.

Foerster, Rolf. 1993. *Introducción a la Religiosidad Mapuche*. Santiago de Chile: Editorial Universitaria.

Guarnaccia, Peter. 1993. Ataques de Nervios in Puerto Rico: Culture-Bound Syndromes or Popular Illness. *Medical Anthropology* 15: 157–1965.

Han, Clara. 2004. The Work of Indebtedness: The Traumatic Present of Late Capitalist Chile. *Culture, Medicine and Psychiatry* 28(2): 169–187.

Han, Clara. 2012. *Life in Debt. Times of Care and Violence in Neoliberal Chile*. London: University of California Press.

Instituto de Estudios Indigenas. 2003. *Los Derechos de los Pueblos Indígenas en Chile: Informe de Programa de Derechos Indígenas*. Universidad de la Frontera Temuco: Lom Ediciones.

Kirmayer, Lawrence. 1988. Mind and Body as Hidden Values in Biomedicine. In: M. Lock & D.R. Gorden (eds.), *Biomedicine Examined*. Dordrecht: Kluwer Academic Publishers, pp. 57–93.

Kristensen, Dorthe Brogård. 1999. Chile. In: *The Indigenous World 1998–1999*. København: Iwgia, pp. 121–124.

Kristensen, Dorthe Brogård. 2000. Chile. In: *The Indigenous World 1999–2000*. København: Iwgia, pp. 142–148.

Kristensen, Dorthe Brogård. 2001. Chile. In: *The Indigenous World 2000–2001*. København: Iwgia, pp. 161–167.

Leder, Drew. 1990. *The Absent Body*. Chicago and London: Chicago University Press.

Lindhardt, M. 2012. Power in powerlessness: a study of Pentecostal life worlds in urban Chile (Vol. 12). Brill.

Lock, Margaret. 1993. Cultivating the Body: Anthropological and Epistemologies of Bodily Practices and Knowledge. *Annual Review of Anthropology*. 1993: 133–155.

Lock, Margaret & Nancy Scheper-Hughes. 1990. A Critical-Interpretive Approach in Medical Anthropology: Rituals and Routines of Discipline and Dissent. In: T.M. Johnson and C.F. Sargent (eds.), *Medical Anthropology, Contemporary Theory and Method*. Westport: Praeger Publishers, pp. 47–72.

Low, Setha. 1994. Embodied Metaphors: Nerves as Lived Experience. In: Thomas Csordas (ed.), *Embodiment and Experience*. Cambridge: Cambridge University Press, pp. 139–162.

Mallon, F.E. 2005. *Courage tastes of blood: The Mapuche community of Nicolás Ailío and the Chilean state, 1906–2001*. Duke University Press.

Merleau-Ponty, Maurice. 2002. *Phenomenology of Perception*. London and New York: Routledge.

Pérez, Gabriela. 2000. Población Mapuche en Chile. Situación sociodemográfica. Censo de 1992. In: Sandrá Pérez Infante (ed.), *Pueblo Mapuche: desarollo y autogestón. Análisis y perspectives en une sociedad pluricultural*. Conception: escaparate Ediciones, pp. 61–79.

Salazar, Gabriel & Julio Pinto. 1999. *Historia contemporánea de Chile II: Actores, identidad y movimiento*. Santiago: LOM Ediciones.

Scheper-Hughes, N. 1994. Embodied Knowledge: Thinking with the Body in Critical Medical Anthropology. In: Robert Borofsky (ed.), *Assessing Cultural Anthropology*. New York: McGraw-Hill, pp. 229–241.

Scheper-Hughes, Nancy & Margaret Lock. 1987. The Mindful Body: A Prolegomenon to Future Work in Medical Anthropology. *Medical Anthropology Quarterly* 1(1): 6–41.

Sontag, Susan. 1991. *Illness as Metaphor: Aids and its Metaphors*. London: Penguin Books.

Taussig, Michael. 1980. *The Devil and Commodity Fetishism in South America*. Chapel Hill: The University of North Carolina Press.

Taussig, Michael. 1992. Reification and the Consciousness of the Patient. In: Michael Taussig (ed.), *The Nervous System*. New York and London: Routledge, pp. 83–111.

Torri, Maria Costanza. 2012. Intercultural Health Practices: Towards an Equal Recognition Between Indigenous Medicine and Biomedicine? A case study from Chile. *Health care Anal* 20: 31–49.

CHAPTER 6

Uncanny Memories, Violence
and Indigenous Medicine

Not a leaf stirs in Chile without me moving it.
(General Augusto Pinochet 1981, cited in Collier and Sater 2004: 359)

On 11 September 1973, General Augusto Pinochet and his junta replaced the democratically elected government of Salvador Allende with a military regime. This regime lasted until 1990, when democracy was again introduced in Chile. What happened during these years, especially to the political opponents of the military regime, is a subject that has only recently been discussed publicly in Chile. The topic of state violence became part of a public discussion in connection with the publication of a governmental report on 28 November 2004, which was written on the basis of 35,000 testimonies given to the Comisión Sobre Prisión Política y Tortura (Commission on Political Imprisonment and Torture). This report documented the widespread violence carried out during Pinochet's

This chapter is a revised version of the following publication: Dorthe Brogård Kristensen 2010 "Uncanny Memories, Violence and Indigenous Medicine in Southern Chile." In *Remembering Violence: Anthropological Perspectives on Intergenerational Transmission*. Nicolas Argenti and Katharina Schramm, eds. Pp. 63–82. New York: Berghahn.

© The Author(s) 2019
D. B. Kristensen, *Patients, Doctors and Healers*,
https://doi.org/10.1007/978-3-319-97031-8_6

151

military regime,[1] especially in connection with the Mapuche, who were often regarded as left-wing sympathizers due to their fight for collective land rights. The report sent shock waves through Chilean society, as many people had previously regarded state violence as an impossibility (Stern 2006a, b; Borzutsky and Oppenheim 2006). Even now, in everyday conversation, this violence is very rarely directly verbalized, and has often been referred to as "the black hole in the collective memory of the Chileans".

This chapter explores the relationship between the medical practice of the machis and issues relating to memory and violence. What happens to experiences of violence that have not been verbalized directly? Are they ever effectively forgotten, or are they carried within the individual mind or the individual body? Are they transmitted and reworked through the social framework and bodily practices available in a given context? Exploring a case study of illness, I argue that memories of violence are articulated and negotiated through the social framework available in a given context, in this case personal narrative, bodily symptoms and indigenous medical practices. A diagnosis—or an idiom of distress (Nichter 1981)—can be considered a language and even a form of life (Antze 1996: 6). Medical practices and disease categories might serve to articulate, confront and rework situations of terror and the threat of personal destruction in connection with memories of state violence. This happens because, through medical practices, the body acquires the vocabulary, images and agency necessary for expressing and negotiating feelings and experiences of terror and destruction.

Consequently, the overall argument of this chapter is that in a context of medical pluralism—in this case biomedicine and Mapuche shamanistic healing—the patients negotiate social positions and collective memories; that is, in illness stories and indigenous healing practice, certain memories and values, olvidos (or hidden) in public discourse, are highlighted and made visible in a parallel form through the use of metaphors (Johnson 1987; Kirmayer 1992, 1996, 2000; Low 1994) and images (Halbwachs 1992; Taussig 1987). In the two previous chapters, I explored the notion of olvidos in relation to the creation of divisions based on class and

---

[1] As a consequence, in November 2004 the former president, Ricardo Lagos, officially recognized the responsibility of the government for the violation of human rights during the military regime (*La Nación*, 29 November 2004).

ethnicity; in this chapter, I turn to the olvido pertaining to experiences of personal destruction and violence. I argue that indigenous medicine is a useful tool for people's articulation and negotiation of a repressed past and a means to change their perception and agency. More specifically, I show how a Mapuche diagnosis and treatment of susto (soul fright) or mal (sorcery) provides a framework for renegotiating the past, especially the traumatic past.

According to Mapuche cosmology, there is no separation between mind and body. The individual body is considered an open entity, strongly connected to and influenced by the social order. An illness is thought to affect the spiritual, physical and social aspects of a person's being; in other words, emotions, physical organs and social relations are all interdependent. As a consequence, it is believed that an incident in a person's present (or past) may affect his or her own well-being, as well as the well-being of his or her social relations; through healing practices, however, it is possible to re-enact and resolve events of the past (Bacigalupo 2001: 42–43; Citarella et al. 1995).

Another important piece of information that comes to the fore in illness stories and Mapuche healing practice is the role that spirits play in memory and in medical practice. According to Michael Lambek, Malagasy spirits are a vehicle for history and examples of a collective historical memory; he adds that "they bring forward and force people to acknowledge the commitments of and to the past. The past is never completely over; it continues to shape the present, even as it is distinct from it, and at the same time is available to be addressed by the present. Conversely, remembering entails engagement with the past" (Lambek 1996: 243). Consequently, a diagnosis involving the presence of spirits can be regarded as a living and embodied history that permits the patient to negotiate his or her relation to the world in images and metaphors, which in turn allows for the reworking of a situation. Therefore, Mapuche healing practice can be considered an act of remembering through the body, and also a way to negotiate past memories and present problems. In other words, metaphors play a crucial role as a way to open the doors to the past and, through this, to negotiate the individual's relationship to the world. Metaphors shape and form bodily experiences, but they also allow the patient to negotiate and act upon a social reality by providing ways of acting upon a representation, and simultaneously sharing the representation with others (Kirmayer 1992: 335).

REMEMBERING AND FORGETTING: A CULTURE OF FEAR

In contemporary everyday life in Chile, the Pinochet regime, notwithstanding the widespread repression and violence for which it was responsible, is very rarely mentioned. The historian Steve Stern, who writes about the memory struggle over Chile's past, provides some astonishing figures. In a country of 10 million people in 1973, individually proven cases of death or disappearance by state agents amounted to 3000, documented political arrests 82,000 and persons exiled 200,000. Torture estimates range between 100,000 and 400,000. These figures indicate that the majority of Chilean families have a relative, friend or acquaintance who has been affected by some kind of violence and repression (Stern 2006a, b: xxi).

The politics of the military regime also had a profound impact on the mental health of the people, firstly because many suffered severe health problems due to torture. Before the military coup, community leaders, psychiatrists, social workers and epidemiologists addressed psychosocial problematics in community mental health. This ceased abruptly at the start of the military regime, to be replaced with hospital-based medicine that largely relied on the use of pharmaceuticals in the treatment of mental disorders (Han 2012: 170). The literature documenting the status of mental health in Chile during the military regime is scarce and mostly consists of studies conducted by human rights groups. Following the military coup, a number of human rights organizations cooperated with religious bodies to provide voluntary health services to persons suffering from mental problems caused by political suppression. The largest organization was El Comité de Cooperación para la Paz (COPACHI),[2] founded in

---

[2] A number of programmes followed. Later in 1977, the organization El Fundación Social de las Iglesias Cristianas (FASIC) founded a psychiatric programme; in 1979, the programme PIDEE (Fundación para la Protección de la Infancia Dañada por los Estados de Emergencía) was established for the treatment of children. Furthermore, in 1980, El Comité de Defensa de los Derechos del Pueblo (COPECU) was founded, which united left-wing personalities; and in 1982, the programme DITT (Equipo de Denuncia, Investigación y Tratamiento del Torturado y su Grupo Familiar) was created, for the reporting, investigation and treatment of victims of torture and their families. In 1982, El Departamento Pastoral de Derechos Humanos del Arzobispado de Concepción started a programme for medical attention. In 1984, in cooperation with RCT (Centre for Torture and Rehabilitation) in Denmark, a centre for documentation and treatment of stress was developed called CINTRAS. In 1985, Policlínica Metodista de Temuco established a programme for mental health, and in 1988, Instituto Latinoamericano de Salud Mental y Derechos Humanos (ILAS) began to specialize in clinical work for the treatment of "extreme traumatization" (ILAS 1996).

1973.[3] It is very difficult to estimate how many people were victims of political persecution; according to one estimate it was 89,183, but this figure only includes verified cases (ILAS 1996: 90). After the transition to democracy, the area of mental health dealing with the victims of political suppression was accorded high priority. In the creation of the programme PRAIS (Programa de Reparación y Atención Integral de Salud) the work of human rights organizations was officially recognized and included within the national health system. Unfortunately, the programme had very limited impact, as few people actually knew that it existed (ILAS 1996: 136).

Although conversations about contemporary health problems are omnipresent in everyday life, the violence of the past is rarely a topic of discussion, thereby exemplifying the olvido in which an aspect of a traumatic past is socially "forgotten" due to the absence of a social framework to express it (see Chap. 1). Often people related these problems to the economic situation, but hardly ever to historical and political events.[4] Yet when I interviewed patients, feelings of terror and destruction often featured in their accounts of symptoms, whether psychological or physical, which were commonly associated with disputes in the family and seen as resulting from the malign influence of spirits or from witchcraft. In contrast, many of my informants were reluctant to discuss issues concerning the political upheavals of the recent past and the state-sponsored violence that accompanied them. Nonetheless, although I seldom witnessed discussion of the violence of the military regime, many of my informants claimed that during the Pinochet era numerous dead bodies had been found in the rivers or buried in the ground—especially in indigenous territories.

The sharp contrast between the silence surrounding the violence related to government politics, which was rarely described or only mentioned in a very fragmentary and non-chronological way, and the ubiquity and loquaciousness of the public discourse regarding health problems—sometimes of

---

[3] Turning to the literature on mental health and the effects of torture on family structure, similar symptoms appear. Not only do the victims suffer, the entire family suffers directly or indirectly from the torture of family members. In the literature on torture and trauma, family members are often described as suffering from feelings of fear, anxiety, uncertainty and grief (ILAS 1996).

[4] This idea has been suggested by Desjarlais et al. as applicable in the case of Chile, in their volume *World Mental Health*, where they point to a study that has identified three core features of persistent fear among the Chilean population: firstly, a sense of personal weakness and vulnerability and a feeling of powerlessness; secondly, sensory perception remaining in a permanent state of alert; and thirdly, a distorted perception of reality (1995: 199–122).

a quite trivial kind—raises the question of whether the latter has not somehow replaced the former: whether talk about current ill-health might link to memories of past persecution. It is possible that these illness stories are—in the end—not trivial at all, but could provide a key to understanding how people cope with their past and present suffering through the use of medicine and bodily practices. The embodiment or somatization of social ills as lingering illness is often shared within a family or group of victims. This has been described in the literature as the "psychosomatic family", which is also characterized by the presence of strong boundaries limiting contact with the outside world (e.g. "we can only count on ourselves"); its members often isolate themselves, choosing not to share their problems with people from outside their family circle. One might even speak of a culture of fear. These problems are often related to having a family member who has been subjected to torture (Agger and Jensen 1996: 273).

The fate of Chileans during the military regime has mostly been described by external observers. In an article in 1985, Ariel Dorfman compares their destiny to the rural legend of the imbunche, which explains what happens when a child disappears:

> He has been kidnapped by witches, and his captors, to ensure his servitude, break all his bones, sew together the different part of his body and turn his head around so he must always look and walk backwards. His eyes, ears and mouth are constantly stitched up. The creature is called Imbunche. (Dorfman 1985: 17)

Dorfman further describes the regime's total control of public discourse, including the closure of six magazines published by the opposition and the strict censorship of all media, commenting that "this control is as arbitrary as it tends to be at times absurd: a child's dictionary sold on newsstands was confiscated—the censors did not agree with its definition of the word 'soldier'". Again Dorfman called on the metaphor of the imbunche:

> Chileans do not know, cannot know, if today their voices will be overheard, if tomorrow their bodies will be fractured. But even if they are not arrested or beaten up by the police or thrown out of their work, they are, in a way, already like imbunches. They are isolated from each other, their means of communicating suppressed, their connections cut off, their senses blocked by fear. (Dorfman 1985: 17)

I came upon Dorfman's link between the experience of repression and violence and the imbunche creature while I was reviewing the illness stories of shamanistic healing in my notes. Here I encountered a similar metaphorical link between the memory of violence and practices of witchcraft embodied in the notion of bicho. The use of the words bicho and imbunche often overlaps. Bicho, as noted in previous chapters, is the Mapuche word for vermin or an intestinal worm, but also denotes an evil force which, through an act of witchcraft, installs itself in, and is nurtured by, a human host from whom it steals the life force.

The following story of a Mapuche man named Aberlardo illustrates the role that medical practices and spirits play in the negotiation and subverting of experiences of violence. I suggest that the appearance of an imbunche or a bicho might be an example of the "uncanny" in traumatic memory, not in the Freudian sense of fantasy play taking place in the mind of a child, but as a meta-reality through which the patient is provided with a means of action (Argenti 2001: 71). The uncanny is, according to Freud, "something, which ought to have remained hidden, but has come to light". In Aberlardo's story, the bicho plays a crucial role in the management of an illness. The creature has many layers of significance, one of which is that it is used to express an experience of being attacked and destroyed by an external evil force. It is also suggested that it represents an articulation and negotiation of that which has not been allowed a direct verbal expression; in this case, memories of state violence.

THE BEWITCHED BODY: THE NARRATIVE OF A SURVIVOR

Aberlardo identified himself strongly as Mapuche; he had been raised in the countryside and was now a returned migrant from the north where he had worked in construction, distinguishing himself by being quite successful. He was a leader of the local community and in charge of the construction of tower blocks in a big town near his house in the countryside. Aberlardo began his illness story, which took place some four years earlier, by observing, "I had a serious health problem, but the doctors did not find anything wrong with me." Subsequently he spoke about his bodily symptoms: his stomach had been painful and swollen and, especially in the afternoon, he felt that something was moving inside his belly; he also suffered from lack of appetite and insomnia, going to bed at 9 p.m. and waking at 1 a.m., almost leaping from his bed in fright. When his colleagues and family suggested that it might be a stomach ulcer, he went to the doctor and had an examination which revealed no ulcer; instead, his doctor gave him tranquillizers. Apparently, however, this medicine was not effective in curing his symptoms.

I suspected that Aberlardo believed that the mysterious suffering he described was the result of witchcraft practices that had damaged his body and mind. The clues, signs and traces he let drop before arriving at the narrative climax were of course of a personal kind, but also reflected a framework for articulating a life story which involved the description of bodily symptoms and the work of evil forces upon human life. During these medical dialogues, memories of the past simply poured out. Talking about past bodily symptoms seemed to be a key that opened the door to other memories of the past. The underlying assumption, which stems from the observations expressed in this illness story, is that medical discourses might encapsulate issues that go beyond health problems. The notions of power and identity in relation to social and political processes also seem to be implied. Or, in other words, these stories reflect how people articulate and negotiate their sense of self in relation to the languages available in a given context.

Aberlardo's story is typical of many citizens in Southern Chile who identify themselves as Mapuche or mestizo and who visit Mapuche healers for diagnosis and treatment for afflictions like so-called Mapuche or spiritual illnesses. In what follows I explore Aberlardo's illness story, which, it appears, is not only related to the bodily symptoms listed, but also to its place within the socio-economic context: that is, its position in a marginal but also alternative space to articulate discourses and memories opposed to mainstream discourses on both politics and health.

Aberlardo told me that he had talked about his health problem to a colleague, who recommended that he consult a machi the colleague knew. He agreed and went to the countryside one Tuesday morning. The machi diagnosed him by sleeping with his shirt (*piwuntun*) and by analysing his urine (*willintun*). Her diagnosis was clear. Due to envy of his success in life he had been bewitched by evil (mal); someone who was looking after his livestock had stolen his clothes—his shirt, socks and underwear—and had dirtied them with cemetery soil and then buried them. "So that you will be gone," she said, "after seven or eight months ... but you are already now feeling very bad." Aberlardo said that he had felt terribly ill for two months and that his father-in-law had been looking after his livestock; he therefore suspected that his father-in-law had performed the act of witchcraft. In Aberlardo's case this was a clear example of sorcery, the result of the conscious intention of the envious other: of human agency.

The machi and Aberlardo agreed to continue treatment, as he said that he "wanted to continue living and knew that [without treatment] he had only five months left". He also wanted to prove "that the power of Good is greater than the power of Evil". The machi gave him a strong medicine made of herbs—an antidote to witchcraft—to make him vomit up the "thing" that was growing inside him. He was instructed to drink it while facing the sun, making the sign of the cross and praying that he might benefit from the medicine. After 15 minutes he reacted strongly, his stomach began to make sounds, his vision became blurred and he saw everything upside down. Afterwards he had to go to the toilet and his stomach started to swell even more. Then he vomited violently. The sight of the thing was devastating to Aberlardo. He described it as "pure, egg-white, with eyes; that means they had black points. That was what was inside me, this bicho."

EMBODIED MEMORIES, ILLNESS AND METAPHORS

In *Beyond the Pleasure Principle* (1928), Freud writes about the way that past painful events seem to repeat themselves against the will of the survivor. While the victim might not have an acute memory of a painful event, the incident is sometimes repeated in dreams and through involuntary actions. Freud claimed that the reason why violent incidents are apparently often erased from the conscious mind is not so much that they have been forgotten, but rather that the victim was never fully conscious when they took place. "The person gets away apparently unharmed" (Caruth 1995: 7), which means that the experience is not fully assimilated at the time it occurs. Only in the repetition—through dreams, thoughts and actions—is the survivor presented with the possibility of actually experiencing the traumatic scenes. Freud observes how the memory of the past often returns in peculiar and "uncanny" ways (1919).

With his use of the term "uncanny" (*unheimlich* in the original German), Freud is not referring to something alien, but to the opposite of *heimlich* (homely), something that is familiar and long established, but that has become alienated through the process of repression. The analysis of the "uncanny" leads, as he says, back "to the old animistic concept of the universe" (Freud 1955: 240), which involves, among other things, a view of the world as inhabited by spirits, where "magical power" is attributed to persons and things outside of oneself. The experience of the uncanny is often related to death and dead bodies, and to spirits and ghosts. Another example is the dream of the "haunted" house or the fear that even an intention can do harm, where certain signs are seen as proof that an intention has the potency to damage. The feeling of the "uncanny" corresponds, according to Freud, to a stage in childhood and among primitive men (Freud 1919), arising in situations where deeply repressed material or the animistic attitudes of childhood are stimulated (Ellenberger 1970: 529). That is, the notion of the "uncanny" is relegated to a realm of fantasy, of children and primitive men, which is clearly separated from reality.

While psychoanalysis would see the past as something that works on us through incidents buried in the unconscious, an alternative version is one that rather locates memories in embodiment and as part of a collective and cultural framework for memory. From this perspective, the "uncanny" is not viewed as something happening in the "mind", as Freud would suggest, but as a living and embodied memory that permits the subject to negotiate his or her relations with the world. Through bodily practices the subject is allowed to negotiate an experience of violence and destruction. Thus, rather than taking trauma as an experience on a merely individual level, it is also understood as part of a society's memory of traumatic incidents that cannot be shared publicly. According to Jeffrey Alexander, cultural trauma occurs when the "members of a collectivity feel they have been subjected to a horrendous event that leaves indelible marks upon their group consciousness, marking their memories forever and changing their future identity in fundamental and irrevocable ways" (Alexander et al. 2004: 1). For a cultural trauma to exist publicly, however, a collective framework for recognizing it as such is necessary. Ariel Dorfman's suggestion of a link between the legend of the imbunche and the destiny of the Chileans is actualized in Aberlardo's illness story, where the imbunche or bicho plays a crucial role as a metaphor for experiences of destruction or violence. In this way the bicho in Mapuche medical practice becomes a way to articulate past violence and a means to rework and transform an experience of subordination. In line with other authors (Argenti 1998, 2001; Kirmayer 1992, 2000; Taussig 1987), I argue that ritual practices might serve to mobilize a memory of oppression, terror and violence in order to transform and subvert it.

DEFEATING THE BICHO, DEFEATING THE VIOLENCE

According to Aberlardo, the machi touched the bicho with a Christian cross and a leaf of canelo, a known antidote to witchcraft; however, the thing did not perish. The machi then had to cook the bicho with medicine to combat and destroy its power. She told him that this thing had been eating him from inside, and that luckily it had not entered his blood, because when that happens, the person is done for. She then gave him some different medicine and said that it would make him sleepy. After half an hour he vomited again and then fell asleep. It was 8.30 a.m. When he woke it was 4 p.m. Then the machi gave him a massage with a Peruvian ointment and medicinal plants and told him to leave the mixture on his body for three days. She served him a soup and asked him how he was feeling. He noticed that he felt as if someone had uncovered his head, as though the weight he had felt inside, like a block of concrete or iron, had vanished. He had recovered and survived; with the help of his friend and the machi, he had prevented his journey to the afterworld. According to Aberlardo, all his troubles had ended. "From then on, I have had faith," he stated, as he finished the first part of his story.

This was, however, not at all the end of his story as a whole. When I asked his family about their experiences, they revealed that the suffering had not only been located inside Aberlardo's body. They had also heard steps in the house and someone knocking on the door, but when they looked, no one was there. They had returned from the north to fulfil their dream of going back to live peacefully in their place of origin, but it had not materialized. The "bicho of envy", as Aberlardo termed it, was growing, not only in his body, but in his house and family and even among their neighbours. They lived together with Aberlardo's wife's family, drinking, arguing and fighting; at one stage the violence became too much—according to Aberlardo's wife—and she left the house for some time. But the community was also haunted by other violent memories; it was as though they went hand in hand with one another. One day, to my surprise, Aberlardo told me that he had just added the testimony of his experiences during the Pinochet regime to the governmental report.

Aberlardo remembered that his father was arrested by 15 soldiers on 26 January 1974. The then 11-year-old Aberlardo hid in a hole, observing the house, the forest, the riverside. A soldier discovered him and told the *capitán* that there were no communists there, only children, but there was no mercy. Aberlardo was put on a red truck together with ten brothers and sisters, the youngest so small he could not yet walk. They spent 15 days in prison without food, forced to witness the torture of their father. His father, however, survived, "only because the old ones at that time were so tough". The children were not tortured, one of the soldiers having said that if they were hit with a club they would die, but Aberlardo lost a brother due to the harshness of the prison conditions. "In the end, we were so lucky," Aberlardo claimed. "It would have been so easy just to kill us, because we were not registered; we did not have any identity papers. They could have killed us and it would have happened as silently as when a leaf falls from a tree. Only Aragua [his brother] fell silent. Only because God is so great did we survive."

This did not mark the end of the suffering, however. Some years later, Aberlardo met a man with white hair and recognized his father's torturer. He was ill for a month after this. In addition, neighbours went missing for months at a time. Parents told their children "This person has committed suicide", but the children wondered how this could have happened as they knew that the person had been arrested: "This happened to Seguel and Don Pedro Millaleo, young guys, not even 30 years old. They killed them and then hung them up near their houses, so it happened around here. If this river could speak and this yard, if you uncovered these places, you could find so many dead bichos here." Aberlardo directly linked his illness narrative with his articulation of the political reality of the Pinochet era. He might not have been aware of having made the link, but metaphorically he used the same expression—bicho—for the "thing" inside his body, the current tensions between people in his family and the corpses of his dead neighbours.

As noted above, a bicho is also known as an imbunche, a small four-legged animal or monstrosity. Even prior to the atrocities of the Pinochet era, the terms referred to people who were said to have been abducted by witches, often as children, and who had been tortured and deformed and thereby transformed into a combination of a human being and an animal. First the witches break the left leg and they bend it over the victim's back, so that it has to walk by jumping, then they turn the head and destroy all the openings except the mouth. The imbunche is created alone, naked, in a cave, where it never hears a human voice and therefore never learns to speak. It is fed on human flesh, often from buried bodies in cemeteries, whereby it can reincarnate through the spirits of the dead and thus increase its power. Witches and sorcerers are responsible for its nutrition, and the imbunche also participates in the meetings of the witches and assists them in carrying out their misdeeds. For this reason it is regarded as an instrument for revenge and harm and is associated with confinement, monstrosity and the illegitimate manipulation of power (Montecino 2003: 244–246).

While the bicho present inside Aberlardo's body could be treated by means of Mapuche medicine, the corpses of those killed in the Pinochet era were much more difficult to deal with. In Aberlardo's words:

The people went to the authorities to report the dead bodies lying around, the animals would not even go to drink water in the river due to the bodies. These people were beaten to a pulp [*sacaron la mugre*]. There were six of them. We went to fetch the livestock and suddenly the horses became frightened, we found four persons, who were not yet dead; they were completely dirty, a lady with a white apron and a man with a tie. The soldier showed the bodies to the people around and from our hiding place we heard him say: "This will happen to you, if you report it."

According to Aberlardo and his wife, the spirits of the dead still caused trouble for the community; often I heard that parents forbade their children to play after sunset or to laugh out loud, to prevent them from attracting unfriendly spirits. On another occasion two mestizo sisters explained more about this belief to me, which they referred to as the phenomenon of the *almas errantes*, the wandering souls. These were the souls of the deceased who for some reason had not crossed the border to the afterlife, some because of their misdeeds, others because they had died violently. Instead of going to heaven, these souls wandered around lost in a vast place between heaven and hell, occupying themselves with haunting living beings: touching them, moving things or perhaps even entering their bodies. These souls could also assist sorcerers and witches in carrying out their evil acts. The sisters told me about a place on the highway where these souls gathered. This was also a place full of crosses in memory of those who had died in car accidents. I also heard many other people talking about the spirits of the dead; one example was the *witranalwe*, the horseman wearing a hat and poncho mentioned in earlier chapters. People told me that the sight of this spirit could result in misfortune, sickness and even death.

These lost souls could be seen as an example of a "living history". Based on his fieldwork on the island of Mayotte and in northwest Madagascar, Michael Lambek argues that spirits are a vehicle for history and examples of a collective historical memory. He writes, "Spirits wear the clothing of the time when they were alive, speak the languages of the past, embody past habits, customs, and comportment; they continue to enact the concerns, relationship, and perspectives of the past" (Lambek 1996: 243). Therefore, rather than mere recollections, the spirits are active remembrances: they link past experience with present misfortune and illness (ibid.). They represent a connection with the past, becoming the vehicle for the expression of this past through the human body.

Aberlardo himself saw his illness as connected to the spirit world; he had experienced problems with spirit presences in the house and his family heard knocking and footsteps, which were related to his illness. Moreover, he metaphorically connected past and present by using the same term—bicho—to refer to the thing inside his body and the corpses he saw in his childhood. Could the bicho in his stomach be seen as an example of something which ought to have remained hidden but which came to light? Whether this is the case or not, it seems clear that it gave past suffering a tangible form that could be treated with an antidote; with the medicine of the machi, he was able to vomit the thing up and to destroy its malign power over him.

THE BICHO: THE EMBODIMENT AND NEGOTIATION OF DEFORMED NATIONALITY

In Aberlardo's case, medical diagnosis and metaphors both played crucial roles in negotiating his past experiences. As noted by James Fernandez (1986) and Lawrence Kirmayer (1998, 2000), the metaphor occupies an intermediate ground between embodied experience and the narrative structure of plots, myths and ideologies, and can be considered the primary way in which individuals and cultures make sense of the world. Kirmayer further argues that metaphors are embodied; that is, they are grounded in the body while at the same time providing it with the ability to extend into the social world. Through metaphor it is possible to move from the abstract and inchoate of lived experience to the concrete and easily graspable. While experiences of extreme violence may not be integrated into the conscious awareness of the victims and the witnesses, images of violence may be absorbed into metaphors in indigenous healing practice.

Michael Taussig calls this "implicit" social knowledge, giving as examples the images of unquiet and spiteful spirits of those who have died a violent death. Is it possible, he asks, that an image impressed in the memory of an individual struck down by violence could exist as an unquiet, spiteful soul roaming the earth forever (Taussig 1987: 373)? Might the spirits of wekufe and bicho in Mapuche medical practice exemplify experiences of violence which society could not contain consciously, but which reappear in uncanny ways? These metaphors provide a framework for action and performance and a tool for working with experience: expressing something that the body is not only victimized by, but also may confront and deal with; communicating something that cannot be expressed openly (Low 1994: 143).

Mapuche healing practices dealing with spiritual illness certainly provided Aberlardo with a sense of agency. After this illness episode, as noted above, Aberlardo and his wife found signs of witchcraft in the house they shared with her family. He then returned to the machi with soil from the yard, in which she found the remains of human bones; she added that someone had also buried a blouse and hair beneath the floor. After this incident, Aberlardo and his wife decided to live on their own and make a fresh start. They constructed their new house on a plot nearby with all new materials. Nothing from the old house could be reused. Here, a new and peaceful life started. They grew medicinal plants in their garden, and Aberlardo regained the strength to struggle for his culture, as he put it, by defending indigenous traditional values and territory. He explained how many of his neighbours have been subjected to violence from the police, due to their claiming of indigenous land, even today. He regarded this fight as part of a general struggle between good, indigenous and spiritual values, and external evil forces trying to destroy these values. Thus, the diagnosis and treatment not only assisted Aberlardo in recovering from his affliction, but also served to embody and strengthen his social values and his sense of the world as consisting in good, positive spiritual forces and damaging, harmful forces, thereby influencing his approach to everyday life.

Aberlardo's illness story can be regarded as an example of what Michael Taussig calls "history as sorcery" (1987: 366): an experiential appropriation of the past that incorporates historical and meta-reality sensitive to the existence of forbidden images. Might the bicho in the stomach be an embodied image from the past? A way in which the past silently afflicts those who cannot speak of it but, by the same token, a way for its victims to manage what cannot be said in another way? A sort of dialectical image, through which the effects of the past are made available to experience?

With the metaphorical link that Aberlardo makes between the dead corpses and the "thing" inside him, this does not seem impossible. The bicho might be an embodiment of the past that continues to act, providing a door to the past and a means of bearing witness to traumatic experiences. If this is so, Mapuche medical practice can be considered an act of remembering through the body, a way to negotiate the past. According to Merleau-Ponty (2002), the body can symbolize existence, because it realizes it and its actuality. On the one hand is the possibility of making existence passive and anonymous, whereby the body becomes "the place where life hides away" (Merleau-Ponty ibid.: 190). Yet precisely because the body can shut itself off from existence, it can also be the vehicle through which trauma victims open up again to the world. This happens not through intellectual means or an abstract effort of the will, but through a conversion in which the whole body is involved. Through the relationship with the machi and in the course of medical practice, the patient is given the possibility of re-enacting the past and identifying him- or herself as an actor who can deal with malign and negative beings, and not as a victim who is acted upon and destroyed (Argenti 1998, 2001; Jackson 2002). Aberlardo's story is in many ways the narrative of a survivor of state oppression, the metaphor for a national identity that has been deformed and destroyed through acts of violence. The expulsion of the bicho had a powerful effect on Aberlardo and appeared to be an effective coping strategy for dealing with distress and bodily symptoms. His story also indicates the further social implications of accepting a Mapuche diagnosis, as it gives him the agency to approach problems in his current social reality, illustrating how images of the past affect agency in the present.

Conclusion

In this chapter it has been argued that illness symptoms—diagnosed as mal and susto—can be regarded as an embodiment of social reality and past violence. More than simply an idiom or metaphor for distress, the embodiment of a social order permits the individual to rework his or her relationship with the world; rather than being subjected to victimization, as the object that is acted upon, the bodily symptoms enable a reworking of a situation. Constructed by local discourse and institutions, they facilitate expressing and acting upon the social context (Low 1994: 142). It has also been shown that by working through metaphor, the Mapuche healing practice permits the patient to recreate his or her relationship to the world. The notion of spirits brings together separate spheres of experience so that shared memories may be negotiated. In Aberlardo's case, it is through the metaphor of the bicho that distinct areas of experience coalesce—dead bodies, envy towards others, a "thing" inside the body—all of which reflect a moral world where the subject easily becomes the object for others. In shamanistic practice and through the relationship to the machi, the patient is allowed to rework an experience of the world. By literally vomiting out the evil inside the body, "evil" is externalized and made manageable, which permits the patient to regain a sense of control and power over a disabling past and to embody those social values that serve to deal positively with everyday life.

The focus of this chapter has been on how Mapuche healing practice works. It is now relevant to identity the frameworks that influence *what* can be remembered and told, and the discourses and regimes of knowledge that shape *how* memories are told. In Aberlardo's case, two factors influenced his illness story: the general focus on illness stories and medical practice as part of Chilean sociality, and the institutional framework of the current government's efforts to collect testimonies of the military regime, which made it possible for him to tell his individual story. When a person articulates an illness experience, it serves as an opportunity to present past experiences within a common framework, and through this to confirm and produce a sense of continuity and community. Yet remembering is more than a mental act; it is also a social act, one that serves to negotiate one's relationship with the world. Mapuche healing practice can be considered a way to remember through action, and a way to cope with both a troubled past and a troubled present. It encourages a joint social framework where the "uncanny", understood as incidents which cannot be shared openly, is given form, generating collective memorial practice and a way to deal with present problems. Through the management of metaphors—in this case the bicho—shamanistic practice symbolically establishes the self as the one who acts, not the one who is acted upon (Jackson 2002). The bicho represents an appropriation of state violence, allowing the patient not only to remember, but also to remodel and transform the experience of destruction (Argenti 1998).

In this case the use of indigenous medicine constitutes a symbol of social position and a resource for negotiating social and power relations. I further suggest that, in the Chilean context at least, medical practices and illness narratives are connected to collective memories of violence through the use of metaphors experienced by the patient as concrete entities. For Aberlardo, the reworking of past traumas was also connected to conscious recall. I would argue that the machi's healing assisted Aberlardo in confronting not only past traumas, but present problems as well. Thus, shamanistic practices are deeply embedded in the social and cultural world and connected with social values; that is, they are resources assisting actors to articulate their present and past and also to act upon the present consequences of past problems.

REFERENCES

Agger, I. & S.B. Jensen. 1996. *Trauma y Cura en Situaciones de Terrorismo de Estado. Derechos Humanos y Salud Mental en Chile bajo la Dictadura Militar.* Santiago: Ediciones Chile America CESOC.

Alexander, J., et al. 2004. *Cultural Trauma and Collective Identity.* Berkeley: University of California Press.

Antze, Paul. 1996. Telling Stories, Making Selves: Memory and Identity in Multiple Personality Disorder. In: Paul Antze & Michael Lambek (eds.), *Tense Past: Cultural Essays in Trauma and Memory.* New York: Routledge, pp. 3–25.

Argenti, Nicolas. 1998. Air Youth: Performance, Violence and the State in Cameroon. *Journal of the Royal Anthropological Institute* 4(4): 753–782.

Argenti, Nicolas. 2001. *Kesum-body* and the Places of the Gods: The Politics of Children's Masking and Second-world Realities in Oku (Cameroon). *Journal of the Royal Anthropological Institute* 7(1): 67–94.

Bacigalupo, Ana Mariella. 2001. *La Voz del Kultrun en la Modernidad: Tradicion y Cambio en la Terapeutica de Siete Machi Mapuche.* Santiago de Chile: Ediciones Universidad Catolica de Chile.

Borzutsky, Silvia & Lois Hecht Oppenheim. 2006. Introduction. In: Silvia Borzutsky & Lois Hecht Oppenheim (eds.), *After Pinochet: The Chilean Road to Democracy and the Market.* Gainesville: University Press of Florida, pp. xiiv–xxv.

Caruth, Cathy. 1995. Introduction. In: Cathy Caruth (ed.), *Trauma. Explorations in Memory.* London: Johns Hopkins Press, pp. 3–13.

Citarella, Luca, et al. 1995. *Medicinas y Cultura en la Araucanía.* Santiago de Chile: Editorial Sudamericana.

Collier, Simon & William F. Sater. 2004. *A History of Chile, 1808–2002.* Cambridge: Cambridge University Press.

Desjarlais, Robert, et al. 1995. *World Mental Health: Problems and Priorities in Low-income Countries.* New York: Oxford University Press.

Dorfman, Ariel. 1985. *A Rural Chilean Legend Come True.* February 18, *New York Times.*

Ellenberger, Henri. 1970. *The Discovery of the Unconscious: The History and Evolution of Dynamic Psychiatry.* New York: Basic Books.

Fernandez, J. 1986. The Argument of Images and the Experience of Returning to the Whole. In: E. Bruner & V. Turner (eds.), *Anthropology of Experience.* Urbana and Chicago: University of Illinois Press, pp. 159–187.

Freud, S. 1919. *The Uncanny* (J. Strachey, Trans.). The standard edition of the complete psychological works of Sigmund Freud (Vol. 17).

Freud, Sigmund. 1919 (1955). The 'Uncanny' [*Das unheimliche*]. From Standard Edition, Vol. XVII, trans. James Strachey. London: Hogarth Press, pp. 217–256.

Halbwachs, Maurice. 1992. *On Collective Memory.* London: University of Chicago Press.

Han, Clara. 2012. *Life in Debt. Times of Care and Violence in Neoliberal Chile*. London: University of California Press.

ILAS, Instituto Latinamericano de Salud Mental y Derechos Humanos. 1996. *Reparación Derechos Humanos y Salud Mental*. Santiago de Chile: ediciones Chile America CESOC.

Jackson, Michael. 2002. *The Politics of Storytelling: Violence, Transgression, and Intersubjectivity*. Copenhagen: Museum Tusculanum Press.

Johnson, M. 1987. *The body in the mind: the bodily basis of imagination, reason and meaning*.

Kirmayer, Lawrence. 1992. The Body's Insistence of Meaning: Metaphor as Presentations and Representations in Illness Experience. *Medical Anthropology Quarterly, New Series* 6(4): 323–346.

Kirmayer, Lawrence. 1996. Landscapes of Memory: Trauma, Narrative, and Dissociation. In: Paul Antze & Michael Lambek (eds.), *Tense Past: Cultural Essays in Trauma and Memory*. New York: Routledge, pp. 173–199.

Kirmayer, Lawrence. 2000. Broken Narratives: Clinical Encounters and the Poetics of Illness Experience. In: Cheryl Mattingly & Linda Carro (eds.), *Narrative and the Cultural Construction of Illness and Healing*. London: University of California Press, pp. 153–181.

Kirmayer, L. J., & Young, A. 1998. Culture and somatization: clinical, epidemiological, and ethnographic perspectives. *Psychosomatic medicine* 60(4): 420–430.

Lambek, Michael. 1996. The Past Imperfect: Remembering as Moral Practice. In: Paul Antze & Michael Lambek (eds.), *Tense Past: Cultural Essays in Trauma and Memory*. New York: Routledge, pp. 235–254.

Low, Setha. 1994. Embodied Metaphors: Nerves as Lived Experience. In: Thomas Csordas (ed.), *Embodiment and Experience*. Cambridge: Cambridge University Press, pp. 139–162.

Merleau-Ponty, Maurice. 2002. *Phenomenology of Perception*. London and New York: Routledge.

Montecino, Sonia. 2003. *Mitos de Chile: Diccionario de Seres, Magia y Encantos*. Santiago de Chile: Editorial Sudamericana.

Nichter, Mark. 1981. Idioms of Distress: Alternatives in the Expression of Psychosocial Distress: A Case Study from South India. *Culture, Medicine and Psychiatry* 5: 379–408.

Stern, Steve. 2006a. *Remembering Pinochet's Chile: On the Eve of London 1998*. Book One of the Trilogy: The Memory Box of Pinochet's Chile. Durham: Duke University Press.

Stern, Steve. 2006b. *Battling for Hearts and Minds: Memory Struggle in Pinochet's Chile, 1973–1988*. Book Two of the Trilogy: The Memory Box of Pinochet's Chile. Durham: Duke University Press.

Taussig, Michael. 1987. *Shamanism, Colonialism and the Wild Man*. Chicago and London: The University of Chicago Press.

CHAPTER 7

The Shaman, the Virgin and the Taxation Authorities

José Caripan is a modern shaman or machi who conducts his consultations in his private home, where he practises medicine based on Mapuche tradition. Today he is considered one of the most powerful and popular machis in Southern Chile and is, moreover, the *lonko* (chief) in the local community. Caripan integrates collective rituals in the morning and the evening into his medical practice and also sees around 300 patients a day (as described in Chap. 3). Known for his precision and spiritual power, he diagnoses through observing the patients' urine (*willintun*), clothes (*pewutun*) or by entering trance. He refers patients to doctors, for instance in cases of terminal cancer or gallstones; however, he claims to be the victim of medical doctors' envy and believes it is very difficult to combine the two kinds of healing. Like many machis, Caripan challenges official discourses of illness and fills a gap in health care that emerged with its privatization and the rise in price of pharmaceutical remedies; this resulted in those people—both indigenous and non-indigenous—who cannot afford biomedical care turning to machis, who offer health care at very reasonable prices (Bacigalupo 2007: 186).

The focus in this chapter is on the relationship between José Caripan's healing practice, the community coalescing around it, and social and political processes. The chapter will, furthermore, analyse his role as an example of the absorption and mediation of history (Bacigalupo 2016a, b), as he mimics and merges the roles of a shaman, priest and medical doctor (Bacigalupo 2007; Taussig 1993, 1987; Kapferer 1997). Don José, as he is called by his patients, integrates elements from the Chilean past to

© The Author(s) 2019
D. B. Kristensen, *Patients, Doctors and Healers*,
https://doi.org/10.1007/978-3-319-97031-8_7

171

become an embodiment of history, a hybrid or bricolage made up from the diversity of cultural materials that characterizes the melding of Spanish colonizers with the native population (Kapferer 2003, 1997; Bacigalupo 2007). Caripan was an orphan (*huacho*), which is a theme that draws on Chilean history, as "huacho" is the name for the many children who grow up in the absence of their fathers (Montecino 1996). He is known for his blue eyes and unusual garb, which consists of a coloured headscarf covered by Mapuche jewellery (*trarilonko*) or a hat, a checked shirt, faded blue jeans and sandals. Among his patients it is widely known that he attributes his healing power to the influence of the Virgin of Carmen, who is both Catholic and the national Chilean saint. Pictures of the Virgin are central in his consultation room and she also plays a fundamental part in his rituals. In his medical and ritual practices, he invokes a Mapuche ancestor and nature spirits, and also uses elements from biomedicine. He connects with political processes in yet another way, however, as he is in conflict with the Chilean taxation authorities, who have threatened to charge him for tax fraud since he has failed to declare the income from his medical work. To his patients this was regarded as exemplifying the Chilean state's lack of recognition of its ethnic minorities. The shamanistic persona and practice thereby imitate the surrounding social environment and historical past, by using them in a healing practice in which spiritual forces play the principal roles.

Caripan's role is central to analysis of how patients project a certain language and form of life into being through medical dialogue and practice which are characterized by stories of the intervention of external spiritual forces in human lives in both destructive/disruptive and positive/ healing ways. Another important feature of his medical practice is the division between natural and spiritual diseases; that is, diseases produced by spiritual intervention. When the illness symptoms are not just located inside the individual body (the psychological regime of knowledge), but also outside in the social body (where the "signs" of spiritual intervention are to be found), the intersubjective and collective participation of the patients is called for. These medical dialogues become an engagement in collective action which moves resentment from a private arena and a private conversation towards the construction of a "counterpublic space" (Das and Kleinman 2001: 10). This popular interest in shamanistic practice in Southern Chile fits the category of what sociologist Christián Parker calls counterculture in Latin America. Parker argues that popular religion in Latin America—in the form of a blend between Christianity and native religion—represents an alternative set of values or, as he terms it, "a contrast culture to modernity" and a counterculture to Western rationality (Parker 1996: 109–111). In the previous chapters I have shown how medical practice is connected to the olvidos of Chile, to the creation of division based on ethnicity and class and experiences of vulnerability and violence. In this chapter I explore the medical work of José Caripan and the medical dialogues connected to it, thereby demonstrating how his persona and healing practice stimulate intersubjective collective engagement on the part of his patients that provides an alternative space in opposition to the Chilean neo-liberal state.

HEALING, COMMUNITY AND SOCIAL AND POLITICAL PROCESSES

This chapter analyses the connections between healing and community on the one hand, and social, religious and political processes on the other, a project associated with the theoretical aim of exploring healing of the individual body in a socio-economic context and the initial question of why people talk so much about illness in everyday conversations. The underlying assumption, inspired by Paul Antze, is that trivial stories, when told in groups, serve to translate shared ideas into experiential realities (Antze 1996: 6). What is important here, as pointed out by Nicolas Rose (1999), is not only what language means, but also what it does and what it enables human beings to imagine and to do to themselves and to others. Language makes people capable of being and doing specific things. Analysed from this viewpoint, stories about illness not only project meaning, but also create a space for action that takes place through healing regimens, tying them to the body and incorporating them into everyday practices (Merleau-Ponty 2002). The illness stories shared in social interaction—the medical dialogues—are not, therefore, simply illness stories, but constitute a meta-commentary on people's social and political reality.

In more classical theories of health, the relationship between healing, community and socio-political processes often remains unexplored; according to Lévi-Strauss (2000 [1949]) and James Dow (1986), for instance, religious healing, shamanism and psychotherapy share psychological dynamics (see Chap. 1). Their aim was to identify the basic principle behind these medical techniques. Levi-Strauss's fundamental assumption was that the shaman and the psychotherapist provide the patient with a language for expressing psychological states and pain. Healing is consequently explained as the manipulation of conflict in the unconscious through the use of myth and symbol, a process which has the capacity to transform individual experience and restore a sense of order. Inspired by the work of Lévi-Strauss, Dow set out to identify a universal principle of symbolic healing, concluding that therapists and their patients operate with culture-specific symbols in a cultural myth. The patient comes to the therapist, who convinces the patient to associate his or her suffering with a symbol that makes it possible for the patient to manage and transform his or her own feelings (Dow 1986: 56). Although these classical theories satisfactorily demonstrate the connection between the disease experience, symbols and healing, they are inadequate to explain why shamanistic healing appeals to people in a specific historical period, as the theories leave little room for historical agency (Fausto and Heckenberger 2007; Bacigalupo 2016a).

Taking inspiration from the work of Arthur Kleinman and Anne Becker (1998) and Lawrence Kirmayer and Allan Young (1998), this chapter argues that the explanation for the shamans' popularity cannot be understood simply by exploring the relationships between the individual body and medicine. It is also necessary to explore disease and healing in relation to power systems, history, and social and political processes. Kirmayer and Becker specifically point to the close connection between morality, politics, the disease experience and medicine. This leads to their talking about a collective body and social memory being expressed in bodily experiences and culturally prominent emotions and categories (1998). Shamanism and spiritual experiences have been regarded as a form of resistance (Boddy 1989; Stoller 1984, 1989, 1995; Comaroff 1985); they have also been treated in connection with the concept of witchcraft and magic as a sort of language that helps people make sense of the world (Geschiere 1997; Petersen 2011). I agree with Bacigalupo (2007: 246, 2016a), however, who notes that machi engagement with different discourses of authority demonstrates a complex interworking of power. Along these lines and inspired by Bruce Kapferer, I am particularly interested in medical practice and social dynamics within the context of a Chilean nation-state that can be associated with the notions of control, regulation and the destruction of opponents. Kapferer (1997) suggests that state power and witchcraft share certain dynamics, and here I demonstrate that José Caripan's healing practices emerge out of a complex interplay with the Chilean state. Furthermore, Michael Taussig argues that certain historical events, specifically those of conquest and colonization, become objectified in the shamanic repertoire as magically empowered imagery capable of causing, as well as relieving, misfortune (Taussig 1987: 367). Indigenous medical practice can thus be regarded as an embodiment of history that both acts within and responds to social forces. Shamanistic healing practice provides a language to make sense of the world, but it also provides a meta-reality, or a model of the world, in which categories, social relations and spiritual characters are used to map the universe.

THE SHAMAN WHO FEARED THE TAXATION AUTHORITIES

I was introduced to the work of José Caripan both through the stories of his healing powers and talk of his strife with the taxation authorities. José and his patients described his medical practice as being in opposition to mainstream Chilean society and biomedical doctors. People told me how he had been subjected to a visit from the taxation authorities due to his refusal to give receipts and pay taxes from the income he received from his practice of medicine. Because of this, people told me, the taxation authorities had threatened to fine him and close down his consultations. Many said that he hardly ever charged for his medical services, which was not quite true, although his prices were reasonable compared to those in the private health-care system. His patients believed that a medical doctor in the municipal council was responsible for José's persecution. Due to these incidents, officially Caripan was not working as a machi, but the stories about him were so abundant that I decided to pay him a visit.

Arriving at his house, I saw a huge sign with the text "No consultations"; this reflected his difficulties with the taxation authorities. Consultation was, however, on offer. A huge, new, two-storey house with a *rewe* (sacred altar) in front, and a flag hanging from the branches of the canelo tree, indicated the residence of a successful machi. I was shown into the consultation room within the house, a large room decorated with rosaries, portraits of Jesus and the Virgin del Carmen, and two impressive silver swords that were used to keep demons away. His consultation was reminiscent of attendance at a Catholic chapel; however, there was no priest here, only a machi. After overcoming his initial scepticism, José Caripan shared his story of the confrontation with the taxation authorities, of how three inspectors had aggressively entered his house threatening to close his consultations down if he did not submit his tax returns to the authorities.

He related this incident to the general tendencies of selfishness and failure to maintain ritual obligations within Chilean society. He also professed to be "traumatized" by it, which threatened both his health and his medical calling to "give medicine to the people". For instance, he had constant nightmares that secret inspectors from the taxation authorities would show up to fine him and ultimately seize his property; his terror was so intense that he believed he would have a heart attack or possibly die of fright. Therefore, he asked that his patients and friends (including the anthropologist!) support him emotionally to enable him to continue to perform his healing work. His well-wishers characterized his medicine as unique, claiming that his medical gaze could see and treat diseases that could not be identified with the technological devices of the medical doctors. José and his patients also declared that he gave the word of God to the people and taught them to behave according to indigenous morality; that is, keeping faith with ritual obligations and respecting nature and all its beings. He invited me to observe his medical practice in order to witness "the power of God" for the people, insisting that I record it to have full documentation.

At this, my first meeting with José, I happened to meet a girl outside the consultation room who, other patients told me, had so much pain in her bones that she had not been able to walk for a week; I heard her shriek in agony, her face pale and terrified. Caripan told me, "Now I will make this girl walk." He turned to her and said, "By the Virgin, stand up and walk." The girl took a few stumbling steps, encouraged by her parents. The mother repeated the story of how the girl had not been able to walk for a week and was in such agony that they had decided to make this long journey to the only one who could save her. José Caripan said to the girl:

> Someone has thrown you negative energy [mal]. Who do you think is your mother? It is not she who has fed and nursed you; it is the Virgin. You must have faith in her; she will receive you, if you believe in her. You need to believe in the Lord; this will protect you against evil.

He then took the girl's hand, squeezed it, smiled and said, "In a moment you will feel a small shock in the heart." The girl smiled and her face started to regain its natural colour; she then sat next to me, still smiling. Everyone looked at me to see whether I had observed all the details of this miraculous cure, which documented the work of the Virgin, *la patrona* of Chile. Through the symbolic use of the Virgin del Carmen, Caripan's medical practice resembles what Michael Taussig calls "history as sorcery". Let us explore in greater detail the significance of the Virgin as a symbol in healing practice.

THE MAKING OF A MIRACLE MAKER

When Don José performs his healing rituals, he invokes traditional Mapuche spirits, the Virgin del Carmen and the Virgin Mary, although the Virgin del Carmen has a very personal significance: in a time characterized by poverty and misery, she showed herself to him and helped him to become a healing instrument of God, a machi, one who brings medicine to the people of Chile. He claims that he often communicates with her, regarding her as the incarnation of the mother of all human beings, the origin of life. I often heard people saying that God and the Virgin have given José Caripan authority and power to provide the Chilean people with medicine to relieve their sorrows, diseases and disorders. He explained his relationship with the Virgin in the following way:

> She helped us. We had very serious reverses, but we prayed with faith. We have so much faith in her, and with her help we always achieve things. … I pray to her and she helps, which is why I believe so strongly in her. I pray to her every night and in the morning I also remember to pray to her, and it is for this reason we are still alive. Without God and the Virgin we are nothing; we come through alive due to their will.

The historical account of the devotion to the Virgin del Carmen is strongly linked to the Chilean people, as, according to popular belief, she was born and raised in Chile, although her name comes from Monte Carmelo, a hill situated in the north of Palestine. The devotion to her began in Chile with the arrival of the missionaries in 1595. In 1817, during the fight for Chile's independence from Spain, the Virgin was presented as the patron saint of Chile for the army of the Andes. On 14 March 1818, a statue of her was raised where the struggle for independence took place and the Virgin del Carmen became the official saint of Chile. The Virgin today reunites the Virgin Mary with the history of Chile. She is considered the country's queen, who does not only concern herself with individual persons, but with the welfare of the whole nation, its progress and development. The Virgin here plays a crucial role as a symbol that unites levels of historical reality and personal experiences of suffering, fragility and healing. She also embodies a Christian morality whereby the world is seen as consisting of a duality between evil/destructive and positive/healing powers; she is a life-giving force and a safeguard against evil.

The Virgin is crucial in the patients' construction of José Caripan as a miracle maker, and belief in her also links to the question of the effectiveness of medical practice and the performance of miracles among Jose's patients in opposition to the destructive forces of social reality. In his house he has pictures of her, and what looks like a Catholic altar to her (Fig. 7.1). Moreover, each year on 16 July all his patients are invited to participate in the celebration of his birthday, which coincides with the celebration of the Virgin del Carmen. This does not appear as a coincidence in the patients' perception of the machi's medical practice, rather serving to connect his spiritual power with hers. The Virgin is the symbol of a historical event—the formation of the nation of Chile—but also a symbolic bulwark against evil, a magic image capable of both causing and alleviating misfortune. By turning to this image, people can reflect on their symbolic potential and hope to manage sickness and suffering (Taussig 1987). To José and his patients, the Virgin unifies every level of meaning and gives hope for a miraculous cure.

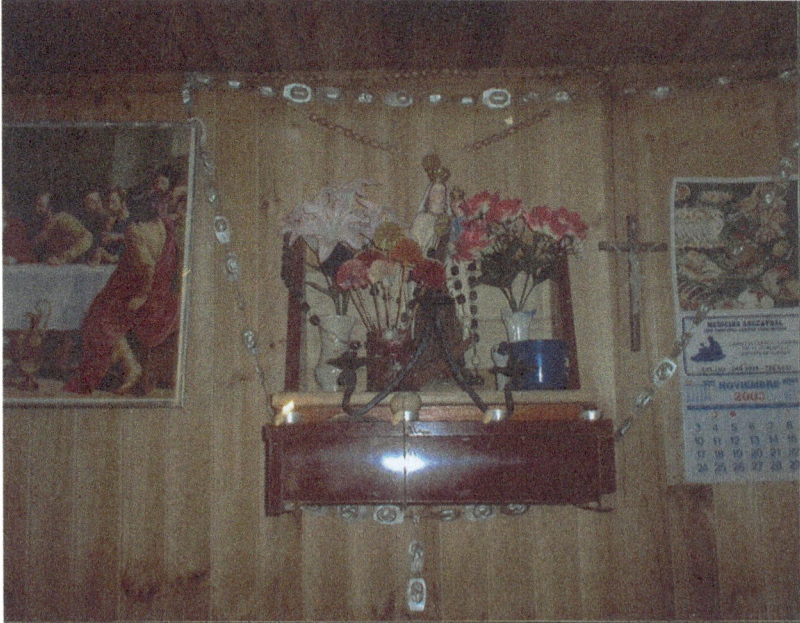

Fig. 7.1   The Virgin del Carmen in José Caripan's consultation room

THE PERFORMANCE OF A MIRACLE

Patients often stayed at one of José's consultation sessions for a whole day, listening to and exchanging illness stories. It was here that I made the acquaintance of many of his patients, later visiting them at home. This section is based on observation of his interactions with his patients during consultation, as well as follow-up interviews with some of the patients, showing how he merges the roles of a shaman, priest and medical doctor. As already described, his house has similarities with a Catholic chapel, but simultaneously it resembles and perhaps imitates the space of a biomedical practice, with a waiting room, a consultation room/office and a room where the medicine is prepared. After examining the bottles of urine brought by the patients, the shaman writes down his diagnosis on a piece of paper (Fig. 7.2), thereby imitating the medical doctor, who also writes down the symptoms of the patient, as well as the prescription for medicine. Once he has looked at the day's collection of bottles of urine, José

Fig. 7.2   The shaman looks at a bottle of urine, identifies the sickness and writes a prescription

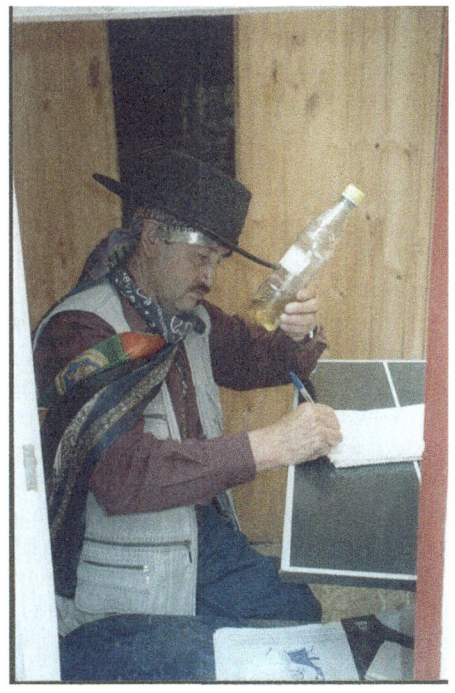

calls out the names of the persons written on them in turn; once identified, he explains to the person what is wrong, and whether he can treat the problem or not. A consultation takes around five minutes. He then gives the prescription to his wife, who prepares medicine from herbs, cooking it up in huge pots in the kitchen with the assistance of two helpers.

While the patients wait for their medicine, they participate in José's activities. Many go to a shelter where a man prepares tortillas at his fireside; here they sit and converse for hours about their symptoms, experiences with medical doctors and other practitioners. In between consultations José might suddenly vanish, to reappear in ritual clothes, removing his hat, placing heavy Mapuche jewellery on his head and taking out his shaman drum. I happened to be present when the 6-year-old Wanglen (whose case study commences this volume) showed up. Her cure was often commented upon by the patients and became almost emblematic of José's healing power. To recapitulate, the girl had entered a state of coma and, after months of intensive medical treatment from both doctors and shamanistic medicine, had finally returned to consciousness. Wanglen's case is interesting, as there was no way to establish which form of healing had cured her, since she was treated simultaneously with biomedicine and Mapuche medicine. However, biomedicine did not receive the same amount of attention as shamanistic practices in the medical dialogue.

A typical day begins with around 100 people queueing up in front of the desk where Caripan keeps the bottles of urine. He picks out a person to help him organize the bottles and to write the names of the patients in a notebook. Other patients gather in front of the bottles, where they greet each other and discuss their health problems. Caripan leaves the consultation room and goes into his private house, where he puts on his ritual outfit; at about nine in the morning, he performs his morning ritual for all the patients in front of his *rewe* against the background noise of the morning traffic. He takes a jug from the altar and throws the water in it onto the crowd; hundreds of hands reach out to receive a few drops of the blessed water, which they use to wet their faces and hands. Then he intensifies his drumming and enters a trance state while covering his eyes with the scarf (Fig. 7.3). His assistant and wife arrive with a bowl containing herbal remedies, which they put on the fire; this produces an intense smell and foggy smokescreen, which mingles with the rays of the morning sun. People gather around the bowl and the smoke and take leaves, which they use to touch their faces and arms. Speaking in Mapudungun, Caripan invokes the spirits:

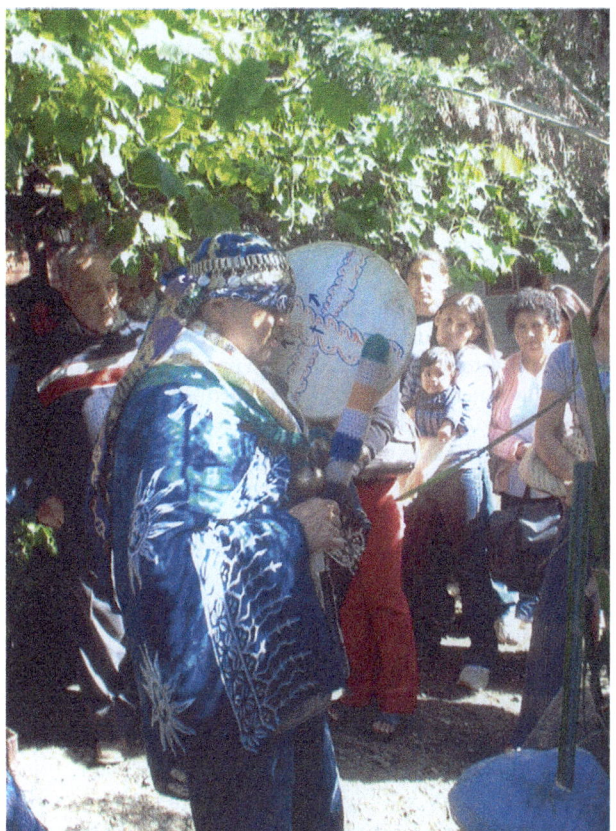

Fig. 7.3 Caripan in a trance during a ritual

We are here united to receive strength, let us unite with hope, let us pray. We are living creatures, for this reason we pray that you look upon us and enlighten us to see what we ought to do. I am only a human being who with your help may realize what medicine to give to your children. Help us to receive your wisdom, and to pray in the correct form for your children who are waiting to receive your food so that the pain and troubles will be eased for those who present themselves at this place.

After the ceremony, Caripan disappears and returns a while later in his normal clothes and starts diagnosing. Between consultations he tells jokes and offers spiritual teaching by turns. The jokes are often a bit impertinent; for instance, if asked by a woman when it would be her turn, he could answer, "Don't worry, I'll have time to make love to you in a moment." This would make the crowd scream with laughter. Then he might suddenly become solemn and switch to spiritual teaching, saying, for example, "When you are praying to the Lord you have to be totally devoted, you have to give yourself with all of your heart. Religion, race and colour do not matter to the Lord." Then he tells the crowd that illness occurs when ritual obligations are not fulfilled. He would explain:

> [The Mapuche religion teaches people] to heal illness by filling a jug with spring water between 1 and 3 o'clock in the morning while calling upon God. This is holy water which can be used to purify the body; this is a source of health, spring water is the water of the earth, it is God's substance, to drink it is like drinking medicine from Mother Earth. You have to understand that we are all children of the Virgin, we are children of God, we form a mental brotherhood. Isn't that right?

"YES!" the crowd would scream back. "We have to fight for love, not for money," he adds. He tells people that so much negative energy exists in the world that it produces illness as well as disorientation in relation to cultural values. He also tells them that he himself is nothing, that he has merely been given the power by God to help human beings to see, act, evaluate and continue their lives. With these words, he suddenly turns on his heel and disappears, reappearing after a while to return to his work of diagnosing.

I am surprised to find Wanglen here in her wheelchair, together with her grandparents, parents and a cousin. Her father says that she is doing very well and so is their work with the state organization of indigenous people. During the consultation, Wanglen's grandmother approaches Caripan and embraces him. Moved to tears, she says to the crowd, "This man cured my beloved grandchild. We thought we had lost her; she was in a state of coma, but now she has returned to us. She still does not walk, but we know that it is just a matter of time." During this scene Wanglen's mother is also openly weeping. A while later I run into Wanglen's grandmother when I am buying a tortilla; she is mingling with the other patients who are sharing their illness stories, and she tells me that there is so much evil and so many evil people in the world. "When life is going well, people start to get envious," she complains.

We talk about Wanglen's medical treatment at the hospital, where they had her on a respirator for two months. However, it was Caripan's medicine that proved effective against the evil of her granddaughter's illness, the grandmother claims, the proof being that Wanglen returned to consciousness the day they consulted him. This was evidence of a spiritual intervention—a true miracle—mediated by the machi José Caripan. I sit down next to Wanglen, who is slowly reading a children's book by pointing to each syllable with her finger. Caripan takes the book out of her hands and starts to read like a child, one syllable at a time; everyone starts laughing, then he says more seriously, in his role of giving hope of recovery from destructive forces, "Wanglen, you are going to be well, you are such a pretty girl, and many people love you." Don José's healing practice did indeed have strong parallels to the healing stories of Christ, meanwhile imitating the language of the Chilean state with his emphasis on miraculous cures being the work of the Virgin. In this way, the story of the miracle of Wanglen is emblematic of the shamanistic technique for creating and projecting a sense of community.

BEING A DEVOTEE OF JOSÉ CARIPAN

Paula, aged 26 and studying education at university, tells an illness story that is typical of those told at José Caripan's consultation due to its highly dramatic and intense use of metaphors reflecting a worldview and moral code based on a duality between evil and good. Paula uses material objects and fetishes in her everyday practice (a cross made by José Caripan and a Catholic rosary), adopted as a result of her relationship with the machi. In Paula's case we see how the use of medicine combined with fetishes became integrated into her own self-understanding and linked her to the other patients and to the social world surrounding the shaman.

Each year Paula participates in the celebration of the Virgin of Carmen and Caripan's birthday on 16 July. She also participates in the rituals he performs in the morning before he starts attending to patients, and gathers with the other patients in the waiting room dominated by the altar devoted to the Virgin Carmen. Paula relates how the machi's healing practice is an instrument of God, and how he has practically changed her life: "Before I did not believe much in the thing with the medicine, to me they were just bottles; so many people are false and make medicine that never works." However, after several of her family members suffered from serious illnesses, the machi became an absolutely fundamental part of their everyday existence. Paula herself claimed that he had saved her from the "voices inside [her] head", which at one point threatened her sanity. She told me about her own illness, which had started after using a ouija board with some friends had resulted in calling up some spirits. One of these had presented itself and recounted very detailed things about her life. Later she found out that the group of girls had taken one of her hairs and used it in a ritual to bewitch her.

After this incident, Paula began to notice what she described as "the smell of rotting cemetery flowers" filling the house; then she started to cry and was not able to move or eat; meanwhile the voices inside her head were humiliating her. Her family took her to a hospital, where she was sent to a psychologist. Paula refused to cooperate, however, as the psychologist had indicated that the voices meant that she had become mad; she recalls how she screamed to her mother, when the staff at the hospital were administering an injection, "Get me out of here, get me out of here," and begged to see José Caripan. Her mother respected her wish and they returned home and phoned the shaman. Some hours later he arrived with a cloth containing two big knives, which he used to combat the negative energies and cast the demons out. He also cleansed the air with incense and burned the pencil and cardboard which were used in the ouija session, producing blue flames a metre and a half long. The treatment lasted for some weeks, with Paula spending the time at home together with her mother, praying to Jesus, listening to Christian hymns and surrounded by objects which José had made for her protection. In these weeks the symptoms did, to some degree, persist, the swollen stomach and the feeling of having an object inside, the constant desire to cry and the strong terror. However, gradually she felt better and after three weeks she returned to normality and to school.

Now she firmly believes in Caripan's healing. As she once told me, "Both me and my mum are now well due to his work; we think his medicine is complementary. My mum is very devoted to God, to the church, and we became very devoted to Don José when things started to happen to us." However, she recognizes that the current health of her family is fragile and must be maintained through daily practices and rituals. For this reason, she continues to attend Caripan's rituals along with other patients who have become devotees, and they always keep things for protection in the house, such as the branch of a tree from the Sunday church services in a Catholic church, a rosary and José's cross made of sticks and red thread, which Paula has put in the doorway of her room. She says that she is very afraid of the many evil people in Chile, who acquire material goods and power through bewitching those more fragile than they. These people make alliances with demons to cause damage, acts, she claims, that are so powerful that they can kill a person: taking blood from a black cat, for example, or putting cemetery soil on the person whom they seek to bewitch. Paula continues, nevertheless, to see a psychologist on a regular basis due to her "low self-esteem"; she believes that it helps her to leave the incident behind and move on with her life. The psychologist also helps her to control her fear that a similar thing might happen to her again. However, Paula believes that the objects that José Caripan has made for her are fundamental in producing a sense of safety against damaging energies. The use of medicine and fetishes, as well as metaphors related to the duality of the medical practice (the smell of rotten cemetery flowers, the fire from burning the bewitched objects), links her individual experience to the sharing of illness stories among the machi's other patients.

The sense of being protected was repeatedly mentioned by patients, as exemplified when Rosa, a 55-year-old woman, describes Caripan's special healing powers: "It makes me feel protected, being near all those things which I know are doing good and knowing that he is doing good things for the people who are watching him." For more than eight years she has been his patient and she often consults him to get herbal medicine for her severe depression, which she combines with the medicine from her medical doctor. However, while she continues to attend her medical doctor and is quite satisfied with him, she strongly believes that José's medicine is more effective than the biomedicine in relieving her symptoms:

> That happens when you know him and his rituals, that is, when you start having more faith. You know that he is not alone, because he has received this special gift from God, who gave him this blessed power. God gave all kinds of plants to his children so they could use them for medicine and for feeding themselves; there exist so many trees and fruits from the ground that we can eat; God gave us on the earth so many things, which we use. And those who have the knowledge of how to use them, they make medicine to secure the health of God's people.

Rosa thus links José Caripan's medical practice with the notion of God as giver of health to the collective community, by framing the machi as God's messenger. Another example of how Caripan is perceived by his patients is provided by Axel, a 38-year-old mechanic and mestizo who was treated by José for a pasmo—a natural disease that affects the head. He finds that medicine and rituals form a strong antidote against damaging influences and social conflicts: "As the machi says, we are all brothers on the earth, we all live under the same sun. We are all brothers, although maybe we have different backgrounds, cultures and languages. I, for example, am Chilean." I also meet Rosario, who is here with her sister-in-law Nancy and is a poor, 50-year-old mestizo woman, who suffers from rheumatism in the legs. She comments on her experience of the ritual:

> I feel such joy. I come there with such a strong belief that I want to improve, that I want to progress; it is because you commit yourself with all of your heart. This day I brought leaves, I immersed myself in the *sahumerio* [incense ritual], I let the smoke pass over my face due to my strong faith, and I raised my arms in my despair because I wanted to improve, and thanks to God and to my sister-in-law I started to walk. ... My legs hurt so much, my knees felt like a hurting substance, but I prayed to God and to the Virgin that I would not stumble. I had felt so alone and in such despair. But when I come here [to Don José's] I start talking to the people—last time I spoke to a lady who had problems with her mother—and I always try to help them, I talk to them. She told Don José about her problem; I was there listening when he said, "Give her a bit of sugar, medical plants and a bunch of flowers; do it with all your faith and your mum will recover." I know of many people there who have been cured.

Among the patients we find Mario, a taxi driver, Paula's father, who tells anyone who cares to listen that Caripan performed a very successful ritual of exorcism on his daughter. Now he is so grateful for her recovery that he has made a service of bringing patients and their bottles of urine to the machi, making use of the opportunity to participate in the service and hear the word of God. Although most of the patients are Catholics or evangelical Christians, they often prefer to go to Don José to hear the word of God.

Most of the patients agree that they cannot do without their medical doctor; however, they are still very critical of the commercialization of medicine, which they claim is emblematic of the modern Chilean state. Common complaints include the cost of medical treatment, as well as the many examples of wrong diagnosis and unsuccessful surgery. One patient tells a group of other patients that medical doctors often leave things inside the body when they operate; another patient of how a doctor wanted to operate on someone's chest for a tumour, but later discovered that the tumour was in the back. Now she no longer attends check-ups at her medical doctor, and only trusts José Caripan. Another says, almost crying, "If we didn't have Don José, then who would cure us?" This makes many other patients nod their heads, saying that they do not trust medical doctors.

Another theme of conversation is Caripan's problems with the tax authorities. One patient claims that Caripan's medicine is absolutely natural, and asks how a modern state can claim tax for the medicine given by nature, by Mother Earth: the trees and plants. Someone else suggests that the problems are due to pure envy of Caripan's success as a healer, and the fact that a local politician is a medical doctor confirms this theory. Yet another patient claims that this medicine belongs to the original people of Chile—the Mapuche—and should therefore not be subsumed by state policies, but administered by the people themselves. Ultimately, the tax difficulty is regarded as a violation indicative of resentment against someone who has been given to the people of Chile by God—to provide them with healing. In one group of patients, I hear talk of the social problems in a small city: two industries are going to close, which will cause massive unemployment. Moreover, the city is known for its many cases of cancer. These problems are linked to damaging negative energies and the patients ask Caripan to perform a ritual of cleansing in their city, thereby framing the illness and social problems there as the products of a universe made of negative, destructive energies, requiring positive healing energies to counteract them.

José Caripan's medical practice offers a worldview and cosmology wherein spiritual, as opposed to worldly, values are central. Yet the biomedical notion of illness is also the background against which Caripan constructs his medical reality, meaning that biomedical elements are not excluded but, rather, incorporated into a single worldview by the division put in place between natural and spiritual diseases. In the case of the latter, the metaphors of "evil" and "damage" which constantly threaten to destroy human lives become powerful tools in people's interpretations of incidents in their own lives. The voices inside the head become signs not of a psychological imbalance, but of harmful, destructive outside forces. Illness itself becomes a sign of an unbalanced society and the moral transgressions produced, for instance, by people's desire to acquire wealth without sharing it with others, or the failure to observe ritual obligations. Caripan's performances of healing miracles become events for activating and reinforcing this idiom, thereby binding patients and practitioners together in collective action. The locus of healing practice becomes an alternative public place for voicing frustrations with the modern Chilean state, but also an alternative space for the collective construction of values connected to providing medicine to "the people".

CONCLUSION: ABSORPTION OF HISTORY, RECONCILIATION AND COMMUNITY

My focus in this chapter has been on the relationship between medical practice and social and political reality. I have used the scenes at José Caripan's consultations to explore why certain actors perceive a certain medicine to be effective. I suggest that José's religious and shamanistic practices provide a framework for an alternative community within the framework of the nation-state. This relationship, however, is characterized by complexity and cannot be reduced to a simple opposition to the state, as the shaman's medical practice largely draws on elements and common symbols that are related to social, religious and political processes and intertwined with the Chilean community. As a result, two poles have developed in his medical practice: the Virgin del Carmen and the strife with the taxation authorities. These are subjects to which all patients can relate, regardless of ethnicity or class; their salience thereby invites everyone into the experience and expression of a collective body and community. In this context, patients perceive Caripan as representing opposition to state power and as protecting them from destructive forces, while simultaneously gaining his spiritual authority through symbols drawn from the nation-state.

Although illness is often associated with social isolation (see, for example, Leder 1990), in this case it provides the possibility to enter a community that centres on the personage of José Caripan. Most of the patients agree that biomedicine is effective against many types of disorder, especially in relation to infections and operations; however, they are highly critical of what they call "the commercialization of medicine", whereby diseased bodies become part of an exchange of goods and money, and subject to market mechanisms. In contrast, José Caripan's medicine is described as non-commercial, as personal, authentic and something that can be trusted. His figure is the focal point of an elaboration of the experience of alienation and social marginalization in Chilean society with which many patients can identify. Clearly, Caripan has created a culture of solidarity, a new form of community and an alternative way of understanding human beings (Parker 1996: 263).

His healing practice serves to embody moral visions which might appear to be both complex and confusing, but, simplified, comprise the statement of a position and of power relations in which patients refuse to be defined as subjects according to the biomedical dichotomy of body/soul. Rather, they have adopted a worldview wherein morality and the fight between evil and good forces are central elements. The figure of José Caripan shows that power need not only be repressive but may also be reproductive, demonstrated by the deployment of symbols of the nation-state as a resource for personal spiritual power (Foucault 1980: 250). The use of indigenous medicine here can be seen as standing for agency and resistance or, in de Certeau's words, an "antidiscipline": an alternative sort of biopower which can be described as a tactic and a "clandestine form taken by the dispersed, tactical and makeshift creativity of groups or individuals already caught in the nets of 'discipline'" (de Certeau 1984: xv). This alternative biopower is, nevertheless, not straightforward resistance to official discourses, but a complex response which also implements national symbols and ideology. Caripan's healing practice provides an alternative to both priest and psychologist, as he offers a coherent, therapeutic, spiritual space and moral universe. Thus, his medical practice represents a counterposition to the state, but it is also intimately tied to its existence.

My insight, emerging from this analysis, is that shamanistic healing practice is so much a theme in everyday conversation among patients in Southern Chile because it provides a powerful tool in ascribing meaning to people's lives through the use of metaphors and symbols that are sensitive to the historical past and socio-political reality. Moreover, shamanistic healing serves as a space for action that deals with the damaging influence of social and political processes. It also serves to articulate aspects of reality which are not addressed directly in everyday conversation; namely, the themes of national identity, social inequality and violence. Thus, José Caripan's healing practice mediates conflicts and gaps and provides an alternative space for the articulation of certain collective experiences within the context of the Chilean nation-state. Ultimately, shamanistic practice offers a symbolic language that dissolves divisions between ethnic groups, social class and religion.

REFERENCES

Antze, Paul. 1996. Telling Stories, Making Selves: Memory and Identity in Multiple Personality Disorder. In: Paul Antze & Michael Lambek (eds.), *Tense Past: Cultural Essays in Trauma and Memory*. New York: Routledge, pp. 3–25.
Bacigalupo, Ana Mariella. 2007. *Thunder Shaman. Making History with Mapuche Spirits in Chile and Patagonia*. Texas: University of Texas Press.
Bacigalupo, Ana Mariella. 2016a. *Shamans of the Foye Tree. Gender, Power, and Healing among Chilean Mapuche*. Texas: University of Texas Press.

Bacigalupo, Ana Mariella. 2016b. The Paradox of Disremembering the Dead: Ritual, Memory, and Embodied Historicity in Mapuche Shamanic Personhood. *Anthropology and Humanism* 41.

Boddy, Janice. 1989. *Wombs and Alien Spirits, Women, men and the Zar Cult in Northern Sudan*. Madison: Wisconsin Press.

Certeau, Michel de. 1984. *The Practice of Everyday Life, trans. by Steven F.* Rendall, Berkeley: University of California.

Comaroff, Jean. 1985. *Body of Power Spirit of Resistance. The Culture and History of a South African People*. Chicago and London: The University of Chicago Press.

Das, Veena & Arthur Kleinman. 2001. Introduction. In: Veena Das, Arthur Kleinman, Margaret Lock, Mamphela Ramphele & Pamela Reynolds (eds.), *Remaking a World: Violence, Social Suffering and Recovery*. Berkeley, Los Angeles, London: University of California Press, pp. 1–31.

Dow, J. 1986. Universal Aspects of Symbolic Healing: A Theoretical Synthesis. *American Anthropologist* 88(1): 56–69.

Fausto, C. & Heckenberger, M. 2007. *Time and memory in Indigenous Amazonia: anthropological perspectives*. University Press of Florida.

Foucault, Michel. 1980. *Power/Knowledge:* Selected Interviews and other Writings. New York: Pantheon.

Geschiere, Peter. 1997. *The Modernity of Witchcraft: Politics and the Occult in Postcolonial Africa*. Charlottesville: The University of Virginia Press.

Kapferer, Bruce. 1997. *The Feast of the Sorcerer. Practices of Consciousness and Power*. Chicago: Chicago University Press.

Kapferer, B. (ed.). 2003. *Beyond rationalism: Rethinking magic, witchcraft and sorcery*. (No. 46). Berghahn Books.

Kirmayer, Lawrence & Allan Young. 1998. Culture and Somatization: Clinical, Epidemiological, and Ethnographic Perspective. *Psychosomatic Medicine* 60(4): 420–431.

Kleinman, Arthur & Anne E. Becker. 1998. "Sociosomatics": The Contributions of Anthropology to Psychosomatic Medicine. *Journal of the American Psychosomatic Society* 60(4): 389–394.

Leder, Drew. 1990. *The Absent Body*. Chicago and London: Chicago University Press.

Lévi-Strauss, Claude. 2000 (1949). The Effectiveness of Symbols. In: Roland Littlewood & Simon Dein (eds.), *Cultural Psychiatry and Medical Anthropology: An Introduction and Reader*. London and New Brunswick: The Athlone Press, pp. 162–177.

Merleau-Ponty, Maurice. 2002. *Phenomenology of Perception*. London and New York: Routledge.

Montecino, Sonia. 1996. *Madres y Huachos: Alegorías del Mestizaje Chileno*. Santiago: Biblioteca Claves de Chile. Editorial Sudamericana.

Parker, Cristián. 1996. *Popular Religion & Modernization in Latin America. A Different Logic.* New York: Orbis Books.

Petersen, Morten Axel. 2011. *Not quite Shamans. Spirit Worlds and Political Lives in Northern Mongolia.* New York: Cornell Press.

Rose, Nicolas. 1999. *Governing the Soul: The Shaping of the Private Self.* London and New York: Free Association Books.

Stoller, Paul. 1984. Horrific comedy: cultural resistance and Songhay possession dance. *Ethos* 11:165–187.

Stoller, Paul. 1989. *Fusion of the Worlds: an Ethnography of Possession Among the Songhay of Niger.* Chicago: University of Chicago Press.

Stoller, Paul. 1995. *Embodying Colonial Memories: Spirit Possession, Power, and the Hauka in West Africa.* New York and London: Routledge.

Taussig, Michael. 1987. *Shamanism, Colonialism and the Wild Man.* Chicago and London: The University of Chicago Press.

Taussig, Michael. 1993. *Mimesis and Alterity. A Particular History of the Senses.* New York: Routledge.

CHAPTER 8

Conclusion: The Control of Medicine, the Control of Bodies

My body is made of the same flesh as the world.
(Maurice Merleau-Ponty 1962: 354)
It would be wrong to say that the soul is an illusion, or an ideological
effect. On the contrary, it exists, it has a reality, it is produced
permanently around, within the body by the functioning of a power …
on those one supervises, trains and corrects, over madmen, children at
home and at school, the colonized, over those who are stuck and
supervised for the rest of their lives.
(Michel Foucault 1977: 29)

By focusing on illness experiences and medical choices among patients in Southern Chile, the overall ambition of this work has been to connect lived experience with social and political reality. The aim of the fieldwork was to explore the management of illness in the context of medical plural-ism, which involved, in this case, medical doctors in the public health system and indigenous healers. Inspired by Thomas Csordas (1994a, b, 2002) and Maurice Merleau-Ponty (1962), the theoretical focus has been on phenomenological lived experience; the book has also explored state power as suggested by Foucault's notions of biopower and biopolitics, or the way that the modern state, through disciplines of the body, regulates and controls the bodies of its citizens, thereby gaining "power over life" (Foucault 1979, 1980). Moreover, departing from the work of Bruce Kapferer and Michael Taussig, a further aim was to explore human agency

© The Author(s) 2019
D. B. Kristensen, *Patients, Doctors and Healers*,
https://doi.org/10.1007/978-3-319-97031-8_8

in the coming into being of the modern subject in the context of a modern nation-state.

Inspired by the insights of Michel Foucault in his book *Governing the Soul* (1999), Nicolas Rose writes that our intimate lives, our feelings, desires and aspirations, seem quintessentially personal. Living at a time in which public troubles seem to be overwhelming, people's mental states, subjective experiences and intimate relationships seem to offer a place to locate their private selves. Rose argues, however, that this belief is profoundly misleading, because personality, subjectivity and "relationships" are not private matters in the sense of not being objects of power; while our thoughts, feelings and actions may appear as the very fabric and constitution of the intimate self, they are, in fact, socially organized and managed in their every intimate detail. Even if it appears as though people govern themselves in freedom, this freedom is also integrated into relationships of power. Rose argues, therefore, that the free, rational, conscious, choosing, autonomous self is a creation of Western capitalist democracies (1999).

Chile makes an interesting case through which to explore the link between private experiences, agency and state power—as described in Chaps. 2 and 3—for two reasons. Firstly, the notion of a capitalist modern state arrived here very late; in reality, Southern Chile did not become integrated into the republic of Chile until the 1880s. Prior to that the Mapuche led a relatively autonomous existence in a nation recognized by the Spanish throne. Secondly, the military regime of Augusto Pinochet (1973–1989) constituted an example of a neo-liberal state where the notion of the freedom of the individual was advocated as fundamental.

The methodological and analytical focus in this book has been on case stories of illness among patients in Southern Chile in a context of medical pluralism. The methodological inspiration came from the Manchester School's extended case-study approach to relationships between human agency, social change, and social and political reality. The modern state and biomedical practices are relatively new phenomena in Southern Chile, which makes it possible to explore the embodiment, the coming into being, of a Chilean citizen in the context of a modern state, in this case through the study of medical practices. As shown in this work, the politics of the military regime were based on the abolition of workers' rights as well as any kind of social security, including health insurance. For one group of people, the lower strata, the abolition of public social security resulted in social marginalization, lack of health insurance and the experience of not being part of the project of modernization.

I have focused on two medical regimens very widespread among patients in Southern Chile; that is, the public health system based on biomedicine and indigenous medical practice. Furthermore, I have explored the puzzle of why actors perceive a certain medicine to be effective. My interest in this question was born from wondering why health problems, often involving symptoms with no apparent organic pathology, as well as unexplainable occurrences in the household, were such a part of everyday conversation in Southern Chile. People frequently referred to these phenomena as "spiritual illnesses" or "Mapuche illnesses" and sought treatment from a variety of medical practitioners, among these biomedical doctors and the Mapuche healers. The underlying assumption, which stemmed from observation of medical consultations, was that illness stories and medical choices might encapsulate issues related not only to health problems, but also to the operation of power and identity in social and political processes. I have here suggested that these local manifestations can be viewed as "culture-bound syndromes" (Simons and Hughes 1986) and "idioms of distress" (Nichter 1981), not understood merely as a manifestation bounded by a culture, but as illness experiences mediated by disease categories, collective experiences and local socio-political reality. That is, the patients' illness experiences and medical choices articulate and reflect power relations and social and political processes. I have examined categories of class and ethnicity as the product of historical interactions between colonizers and native inhabitants. Furthermore, I have analysed how people creatively articulate and negotiate these categories through their medical choices and illness stories. I have also focused on metaphors and symbols that serve to project a certain language into action.

In my work I touch upon the consequences that this analysis has for the existence of a health-care system based on complementary medicine; that is, the co-existence of different types of medicine. What are the power relations between the patient and practitioners who represent different medical systems? What are the possibilities for agency within the social and political reality that they provide the patient? In other words, I have analysed the different medical practices (public health setting, urban Mapuche clinic, rural Mapuche healer) in terms of their mutual relationship with regard to the social and political reality in Chile today.

FIELDWORK AND FINDINGS

My original hypothesis was that Mapuche illness was closely connected to a notion of cultural identity and tied to the struggle to articulate an indigenous identity. I had to revise this at the beginning of my fieldwork, as it became increasingly evident that the field was much more complex; for instance, I encountered many patients attending Mapuche medical practitioners who identified themselves as mestizo. By exploring different ethnic groups and types of patients (who identified themselves as Chilean or Mapuche), I have analysed how choosing Mapuche diagnosis and medicine was tied not only to cultural identity, but also to class relations.

In Chap. 1, I describe my original assumption that through the study of the unit of analysis, consisting of medical consultations and patient cases, it would be possible to explore the relationship between medical choices and notions of power and identity. I therefore designed a plan for my fieldwork where the aim was to follow the patients of four different medical practitioners in a context of medical pluralism; that is, in the public health service and in the field of indigenous Mapuche medicine. This method also highlighted power relations between different types of medical practitioners. While the field of biomedicine was strongly controlled and restricted by state policy and bureaucracy, the practice of Mapuche medicine was not subjected to legal restriction and was, as such, an "open" field to enter. I was thus not entirely successful in penetrating the public health system; although I managed to interview the staff and medical practitioners, I could not obtain the official permission required in order to follow and interview patients outside the institutional setting. My fieldwork in that context was, as a result, restricted to observing patients during medical consultations. In contrast, in the field of Mapuche medicine, various medical practitioners agreed to participate in the study, I could very easily establish contact with patients and both medical practitioners and patients were very accessible.

Chapter 1 also presented the theoretical and analytical background for the study. Theoretically, this work is based on the notion of embodiment (Csordas 1994a, b, 2002) and the distinction in medical anthropology between the individual and the social body and body politics (Scheper-Hughes and Lock 1987; Lock and Scheper-Hughes 1990). I explored the missing link between the notion of the three bodies as different aspects of languages. Firstly, in what I have referred to as "medical dialogue" (Crandon-Malamud 1986), people share illness stories in social interaction. As Paul Antze (1996) suggests, these stories might reveal how major cultural discourses find their way into people's experience and understanding of themselves. Secondly, I have suggested that the language in medical practices and illness stories represents an articulation of social and political processes or a meta-reality. Here a special focus was on the olvidos of Chile, the forgotten collective experiences denied direct verbal expression. My assumption, however, was that in medical dialogue about illness symptoms and medical practice, people uncovered realities that were the forgotten or repressed aspects of official discourses.

I have described and analysed aspects of olvidos by studying a group of actors and different processes related to medical practice. A fundamental observation was that actors do not necessarily make a choice between an indigenous versus a non-indigenous identity, or between a biomedical or a shamanistic disease category; rather, they combine the two different medical practices, as both biomedical and shamanistic categories seem to appeal to them regardless of their ethnic identity—but for different reasons, and as part of different sets of strategies. It is precisely in the interaction *between* the medical systems that patients negotiate their social position. What might seem to be opposed types of diagnosis are in fact complementary in the medical choices of the patients. Furthermore, concerning the question of effectiveness, I highlighted different mechanisms implicit in medical choices by different groups of actors; that is, how medical choices relate to an articulation of cultural identity and social position. Discussion concentrated on two groups of actors well represented in the medical consultations of Mapuche practitioners: women with mestizo backgrounds, and young Mapuche with a history of migration.

ILLNESS STORIES AND MEDICAL PRACTICES: UNPACKING THE OLVIDOS OF CHILE

My underlying argument and insight are that medical choices are embedded in social and political processes linked to the creation of the modern Chilean state. I have presented three types of olvidos—that is, collective forgetting—in connection with the national ideology. The mestizo came to be seen as the ideal, ethnic homogenous modern citizen, part of the ideology of the Chilean republic, demonstrating the ideology of the whitening of the mestizo population (given that the paler skin colour of the mestizo was associated with advanced civilization). Indigenous blood was stigmatized and associated with all that is uncivilized and backward and simply not part of the modern Chile. Instead, a neo-liberal ideology offered a model of the worker's freedom to consume. One of the consequences of this is the officially unacknowledged creation of asymmetrical power relations between indigenous and mestizo, and poor and rich. The class division and creation of a group of poor and marginalized citizens were referred to as the second olvido. A third olvido, or collective forgetting, concerns state violence, the oppression of opponents of the national ideology, most radically during the military regime's torture of its political opponents.

I have analysed how medical choices relate to or are associated with these olvidos by examining diagnostic processes, medical dialogues and medical treatment. Furthermore, I have focused on the role of the "therapy management group" (Janzen 1978) in the diagnostic process in biomedical practice and Mapuche medicine. In Chap. 3, the focus was on the medical gaze in two types of diagnostic processes, psychiatry and Mapuche medical practice. The two categories—the fixed biomedical type with its established list of symptoms, and the indigenous, which is more concerned with causation and the aetiology of symptoms—are part of a field of navigation and provide different frameworks for action. I have suggested that biomedical disease categories appeal in the sense that official approval of a set of symptoms is an inherent element; in contrast, indigenous disease categories are attractive to patients because they open up an intersubjective and social space for the identification of possible causes and signs—and for the making of selfhood. Hence, sickness becomes a "collective moral practice" which also involves the search for signs of immoral acts; meanwhile, the social relations of the patient—the "therapy management group"—acquire a much more active role in the process of diagnosis and treatment.

In Chaps. 4 and 5, I further analysed the diagnostic process with regard to two groups of patients who were dominant in the medical consultation of Mapuche healers; that is, poor mestizo women, and young Mapuche with a history of migration. In Chap. 4, I queried why so many mestizo women preferred Mapuche medicine and diagnosis to the treatment offered in the official health system, suggesting that experiences of mistrust and marginalization related to the creation of inequalities in the health system made the use of Mapuche medicine more attractive. This intrinsic difference between medical systems is a product of the neo-liberal model, which combined private and public health services of vastly differing quality and cost, wherein the poor were assigned long waiting periods, poor attention and lack of medicine and technologies. Mapuche medicine became a solution to this, uniting mestizo women with Mapuche women in a similar (lower) social stratum. The medical choice of Mapuche treatment and diagnosis reflected experiences of vulnerability and the negotiation of social inequalities, leading, through medical dialogue, to the forging of alliances across ethnic borders.

In Chap. 5, the focus was on another group of patients, young Mapuche migrants, who were mainly treated for depression and indigenous illnesses such as susto and *perrimonton*. I analysed the cases of two Mapuche men, both of whom first presented as suffering mainly from depression but, in the diagnostic process, demonstrably integrated several types of illness, diagnosis and treatment. In other words, they also functioned within a spiritual or "Mapuche" diagnosis related to a notion of external forces, as well as notions of sickness tied to morality. Thus, what might seem like confusing and fragmented strands of identity and diagnosis were, in fact, regarded as not accidental at all; rather, this diagnostic process represented referential dissonances and resonances, gaps or matches in the languages and values that informed the lives of the young men. Seen from this perspective, it is possible that the choice of a Mapuche practitioner in an urban setting was a way to mediate these opposing realities and responses, reflecting a quest for a medical treatment practitioner who would constitute a match between personal experience, social environment and sociopolitical order.

It is no coincidence that patients identifying as Mapuche often choose the more modern, urban Mapuche clinic, while mestizos tend to seek the apparently more authentic, rural healer. Both choices reflect referential dissonance, a gap in the languages that inform the patients' lives: in the negotiation of social position, groups cross ethnic borders. However, the range of possibilities for action is not the same for all actors. The experience of illness symptoms and the use of medicine are negotiated in relation to social and cultural categories and the possibilities made available by the social arena. In order to negotiate the stigma of being indigenous, patients may choose the biomedical paradigm of disease; simultaneously, the fixed categories of ethnicity and class are challenged and negotiated in their illness experiences and medical choices, with the latter providing the creative possibility to overturn those fixed categories delimiting the individual's range of agency. Medical choice makes it possible to break the spell of repressed collective experiences and claim agency and personal space for articulation.

I subsequently analysed some of the potentialities that indigenous medical practice provides to patients in relation to notions of the individual body, as well as the collective and social body. In Chap. 6, I presented the case of a Mapuche man who was suffering from witchcraft (mal), exploring the link between the memory of state violence and illness experiences, whereby the monstrosity of deformed nationality is manifested as a spiritual creature, incarnated in the bicho and the imbunche. The bicho is considered both an instrument of evil and a metaphor for experiences of being attacked and destroyed; it is also perceived as a concrete entity which inserts itself into the body of the victim. Therefore, the metaphor of the bicho represents past experiences—in this case the experience of state violence—but it also allows for their re-experiencing and negotiation.

In Chap. 7, I focused on the medical practice of a Mapuche shaman, José Caripan, around whose preaching of Mapuche religion a cult had developed that was also associated with his healing powers. I analysed how his shamanistic practice calls for collective action. When the illness symptoms are not just located inside the individual body (the psychological regime of knowledge) but also outside in the social body (where the "signs" of spiritual intervention are to be found), the intersubjective and collective participation of patients is called for. Therefore, the medical practices and illness stories move the locus of experience from a private arena and a private conversation towards the construction of a collective space (Das and Kleinman 2001). Consequently, José Caripan's medical practice constitutes an implicit critique of the modern state for failing to provide medicine to its people. Conversely, the medical practice, involving as it does all those who care to participate regardless of ethnicity and class, dissolves class and ethnic categories and represents a resolution for the olvidos, the cultural repressions and collective forgetting. Thus, Caripan offers medicine not only to ameliorate physical and psychological symptoms, but also to provide comfort in the social fragmentation and isolation that are the subjective everyday experiences of many of his patients. This breaks with the neo-liberal notion of individual freedom and individualism, meanwhile challenging the statist control of bodies. In that sense, Caripan's medical practice also challenges Foucault's notion of biopower and biopolitics, as it brings to the surface the inherent creativity and human agency of people even in the face of state control. However, as shown, this is not a simple resistance to official discourses, but a complex response which also integrates the use of national symbols. In one way his practice is counterposed to the state, but it is also intimately tied to its existence.

CULTURAL COMPLEXITY: MUTUALLY CONSTITUTING LANGUAGES

What does this analysis say about the relationship between individual illness experiences and social and political reality? Does the presence of magical stories in the lives of average Chileans express some remnant of old traditions in contemporary Chile, or is it perhaps modern precisely because of its hybridism and reinvention of tradition? Overall, the analysed illness experiences reveal themselves as both reflections of and responses to a global complexity of simultaneously opposing forces: on the one hand, the rational forces of the modern state and the modern citizen; on the other, the magical and mysterious, the "uncanny", which Freud identified as a childish fantasy. Here I suggest that this is, rather, a second-world reality (Argenti 1998, 2001), which might be an inherent quality of the modern: the existence of an alternative reality for expressing and negotiating collective experiences that may not be expressed openly in official discourse.

Remembering Nicolas Rose's work on technologies within the modern state that govern the soul, it is interesting to see the range of possibilities that the different ways of perceiving illness provide to the patient. Firstly, there is the biomedical notion of disease as an individual occurrence taking place in the individual body. In this version, the individual has the freedom and choice to improve his or her health situation. This goes hand in hand with discourses of "self-care" and "self-governmentality", where the self is perceived as sovereign and morally autonomous and responsible for his or her own well-being (Han 2012: 5). In contrast, in the spiritual Mapuche version, the cause of the illness is attributed to an external force, that of a witch or a spirit. Therefore, shamanistic practice in some cases provides increased (or alternative) space for agency. When the cause of illness is located outside the individual body (such as in the person of the witch), collective action in order to deal with destructive forces becomes possible. This is perhaps precisely why spiritual diagnosis or Mapuche illness is perceived as appealing even in modern times, regardless of the ethnicity of the patient, as it breaks with the prevalent thrust towards self-care and individual responsibility, instead calling for a collective framework of action. It is here that Foucault's concept of biopower, the discipline and regulations he describes as being a fundamental facet of the modern state, might inevitably and always elicit a creative response from subjects.

MULTIPLE MEDICAL REALITIES: THE EFFECTIVENESS
OF MAPUCHE MEDICINE

A final question, which has been left unanswered, is whether Mapuche medicine is effective as a medical cure. This leads to another question that I have not addressed, namely: How should effectiveness be measured? Due to a lack of data on the actual physical conditions of the patients, it is here impossible to judge whether those participating in this study were cured in a biomedical sense. However, what appears to be clear is that many did experience an improvement in their condition, although this was never fully recognized by the biomedical doctors I interviewed. One doctor sceptically commented that in those cases where the patients had reported an improvement in their condition after being treated by a Mapuche practitioner, they were never ill in the first place; they just believed they were ill because they felt miserable. Another doctor observed that they would most likely have been cured anyway. Still, what could be argued on the basis of this is that for a certain group of people, Mapuche medicine does result in self-perceived well-being; the question of whether Mapuche medicine is actually effective against biological or psychiatric disease remains open.

What this work concludes is that Mapuche medicine is perceived as effective by a large group of patients because it allows for a collective response to collective experiences of the local socio-political reality. In other words, it is based on a reciprocity between multiple medical and social realities, thereby highlighting the link between the perception of the body, self and social change. I therefore suggest that the success of a Mapuche shaman like José Caripan may depend on the fact that his medical practice is sensitive to social and political processes. Indigenous medical practice does not offer a static universal medical reality, but a form of healing that resonates with the needs and experiences of the members of a given society. In that sense, this medicine is also based on collective experiences, rather than only on individual notions of illness. Therefore, I conclude here with my ultimate suggestion, which is that in a multicultural context, medical practice such as the bricolage that José offers might be a necessary supplement to the official form, as it responds to collective experience and identities. It is precisely in the link between the individual and the social body that one of the secrets of the perceived effectiveness of medicine is to be found.

REFERENCES

Antze, Paul. 1996. Telling Stories, Making Selves: Memory and Identity in Multiple Personality Disorder. In: Paul Antze & Michael Lambek (eds.), *Tense Past: Cultural Essays in Trauma and Memory*. New York: Routledge, pp. 3–25.

Argenti, Nicolas. 1998. Air Youth: Performance, Violence and the State in Cameroon. *Journal of the Royal Anthropological Institute* 4(4): 753–782.

Argenti, Nicolas. 2001. *Kesum-body* and the Places of the Gods: The Politics of Children's Masking and Second-world Realities in Oku (Cameroon). *Journal of the Royal Anthropological Institute* 7(1): 67–94.

Crandon-Malamud, Libbet. 1986. Medical Dialogue and the Political Economy of Medical Pluralism: a Case from Rural Highland Bolivia. *American Ethnologist* 13(3): 463–477.

Csordas, Thomas. 1994a. *The Sacred Self: A Cultural Phenomenology of Charismatic Healing*. Berkeley and Los Angeles: University of California Press.

Csordas, Thomas. 1994b. Introduction: The Body as Representation and Being-in-the-world. In: Thomas Csordas (ed.), *Embodiment and Experience: The Existential Ground of Culture and Self*. Cambridge: Cambridge University Press, pp. 1–27.

Csordas, Thomas. 2002. Embodiment as a Paradigm for Anthropology. In: *Body/Meaning/Healing*. New York: Palgrave Macmillan, pp. 58–88.

Das, Veena & Arthur Kleinman. 2001. Introduction. In: Veena Das, Arthur Kleinman, Margaret Lock, Mamphela Ramphele & Pamela Reynolds (eds.), *Remaking a World: Violence, Social Suffering and Recovery*. Berkeley, Los Angeles, London: University of California Press, pp. 1–31.

Foucault, Michel. 1977. *Discipline and Punishment. The Birth of the Prison*. New York. Penguin Books.

Foucault, Michel. 1979. *The History of Sexuality. Vol. 1: An Introduction*. London: Penguin Books.

Foucault, Michel. 1980. *Power/Knowledge:* Selected Interviews and other Writings. New York: Pantheon.

Han, Clara. 2012. *Life in Debt. Times of Care and Violence in Neoliberal Chile*. London: University of California Press.

Janzen, John. 1978. *The Quest for Therapy: Medical Pluralism in Lower Zaire*. Berkeley, Los Angeles, and London: University of California Press.

Lock, Margaret & Nancy Scheper-Hughes. 1990. A Critical-Interpretive Approach in Medical Anthropology: Rituals and Routines of Discipline and Dissent. In: Thomas M. Johnson and Carolyn Fishel Sargent (eds.), *Medical Anthropology, Contemporary Theory and Method*. Westport: Praeger Publishers, pp. 47–73.

Lock, Margaret & Nancy Scheper-Hughes. 1996. A Critical-Interpretive Approach in Medical Anthropology: Rituals and Routines of Discipline and Dissent. In: Carolyn Fishel Sargent and Thomas M. Johnson (eds.), *Medical Anthropology, Contemporary Theory and Method*. Westport: Praeger Publishers, Rev. ed., pp. 41–70.

Merleau-Ponty, Maurice. 1962. *Phenomenology of Perception*. London and New York: Routledge.

Nichter, Mark. 1981. Idioms of Distress: Alternatives in the Expression of Psychosocial Distress: A Case Study from South India. *Culture, Medicine and Psychiatry* 5: 379–408.

Ronald C. Simons & Charles C. Hughes. 1986. *The culture-bound syndromes: Folk illnesses of psychiatric and anthropological interest*. In: Ronald C. Simons & Charles C. Hughes (eds.). The Netherlands: D. Reidel.

Rose, Nicolas. 1999. *Governing the Soul: The Shaping of the Private Self*. London and New York: Free Association Books.

Scheper-Hughes, Nancy & Margaret Lock. 1987. The Mindful Body: A Prolegomenon to Future Work in Medical Anthropology. *Medical Anthropology Quarterly* 1(1): 6–41.

REFERENCES

Agger, I. & S.B. Jensen. 1996. *Trauma y Cura en Situaciones de Terrorismo de Estado. Derechos Humanos y Salud Mental en Chile bajo la Dictadura Militar.* Santiago: Ediciones Chile America CESOC.

Aguirre, S.M., Philippi, L., Artigas, D. & Obach, A. 2003. *Mitos de Chile: Diccionario de seres, magias y encantos.* Sudamericana.

Alexander, J., et al. 2004. *Cultural Trauma and Collective Identity.* Berkeley: University of California Press.

Alonqueo, M. 1979. *Instituciones religiosas del pueblo mapuche: Ngillathún, Ul. uthún, Machithún y Ngeikurrehwen* (Vol. 7). Ediciones Nueva Universidad, Pontificia Universidad Católica de Chile, Vicerrectoria de Comunicaciones.

Anderson, Benedict. 1983. *Imagined Communities.* London: Verso.

Antze, Paul. 1996. Telling Stories, Making Selves: Memory and Identity in Multiple Personality Disorder. In: Paul Antze & Michael Lambek (eds.), *Tense Past: Cultural Essays in Trauma and Memory.* New York: Routledge, pp. 3–25.

Antze, Paul & Michael Lambek (eds.). 1996. *Tense Past: Cultural Essays in Trauma and Memory.* New York: Routledge.

Arana, Diego Barros. 1884. *Historia de Chile.* Santiago de Chile: Ediciones Rafel Jover.

Arana, Diego Barros. 1934. *Origines de Chile: Los Fundamentos de la Nacionalidad.* Santiago de Chile: Editorial Nascimiento.

Argenti, Nicolas. 1998. Air Youth: Performance, Violence and the State in Cameroon. *Journal of the Royal Anthropological Institute* 4(4): 753–782.

Argenti, Nicolas. 2001. *Kesum-body* and the Places of the Gods: The Politics of Children's Masking and Second-world Realities in Oku (Cameroon). *Journal of the Royal Anthropological Institute* 7(1): 67–94.

© The Author(s) 2019   205
D. B. Kristensen, *Patients, Doctors and Healers,*
https://doi.org/10.1007/978-3-319-97031-8

Argenti, Nicolas & Katharina Schramm. 2006. *Violence and Memory*. Position paper presented at EASA Conference.

Aylwin, José. 1995. Antecedentes Historico-legislativos para el Estudio de Comunidades Reduccionales Mapuche. *Pentukun*: 23–37.

Aylwin, José. 2000. Los Conflictos en el Territorio Mapuche: Antecedentes y Perspectivas. *Revista Perspectivas* 3(2).

Aylwin, José. 2007. La política del "nuevo trato": Antecedentes, alcances y limitaciones. *El gobierno de Lagos, los pueblos indígenas y el "nuevo trato"*. Santiago: LOM Ediciones.

Bacigalupo, Ana Mariella. 2001. *La Voz del Kultrun en la Modernidad: Tradicion y Cambio en la Terapeutica de Siete Machi Mapuche*. Santiago de Chile: Ediciones Universidad Catolica de Chile.

Bacigalupo, Ana Mariella. 2004. The Mapuche Man Who Became a Woman Shaman. *American Ethnologist* 31: 440–457.

Bacigalupo, Ana Mariella. 2005. Gendered Rituals for Cosmic Wholeness. *Journal of Ritual Studies*: 53–63.

Bacigalupo, Ana Mariella. 2007. *Thunder Shaman. Making History with Mapuche Spirits in Chile and Patagonia*. Texas: University of Texas Press.

Bacigalupo, Ana Mariella. 2016a. *Shamans of the Foye Tree. Gender, Power, and Healing among Chilean Mapuche*. Texas: University of Texas Press.

Bacigalupo, Ana Mariella. 2016b. The Paradox of Disremembering the Dead: Ritual, Memory, and Embodied Historicity in Mapuche Shamanic Personhood. *Anthropology and Humanism* 41.

Bacigalupo, Ana Mariella. 2018. The Mapuche Undead Never Forget: Traumatic Memory and Cosmopolitics in Post-Pinochet Chile. *Anthropology and Humanism* 43(2): 1.

Baer, Hans, Merrill Singer & Ida Susser. 1995. What is Medical Anthropology About? In: Hans Baer & Merrill Singer (eds.), *Medical Anthropology and the World System: A Critical Perspective*. Westport, Connecticut: Bergin & Garvey, pp. 1–37.

Baer, Roberta, et al. 2003. A Cross-Cultural Approach to the Study of the Folk Illness Nervios. *Culture, Medicine and Psychiatry* 27: 315–337.

Beneduce, R. 2016. Traumatic pasts and the historical imagination: symptoms of loss, postcolonial suffering, and counter-memories among African migrants. *Transcultural psychiatry*, 53(3), pp. 261–285.

Bengoa, José. 1985. *Historia del Pueblo Mapuche*. Santiago de Chile: Ediciones Sur Coleccion.

Bengoa, José. 1999. *Historia de un Conflicto: El Estado y los Mapuches en el Siglo XX*. Planeta SA.

Boccara, Guillaume. 2002. The Mapuche People in Post-Dictatorship Chile. *Ètudes Rurales*. No. 163/164. Terre Territoire Appartenances: 283–303.

Boccara, G. & Seguel-Boccara, I. 1999. Políticas indígenas en Chile (Siglos XIX y XX). De la asimilación al pluralismo (El caso mapuche). *Revista de Indias* 59(217): 741–774.

Boddy, Janice. 1989. *Wombs and Alien Spirits, Women, men and the Zar Cult in Northern Sudan*. Madison: Wisconsin Press.

Bolton, R. 1981. Susto, Hostility, and Hypoglycemia. *Ethnology* 19: 261–276.

Bonelli, C. 2012. Ontological disorders: Nightmares, psychotropic drugs and evil spirits in southern Chile. *Anthropological Theory* 12(4): 407–426.

Bonelli, C. 2014. What Pehuenche blood does: hemic feasting, intersubjective participation, and witchcraft in Southern Chile. *Hau: Journal of Ethnographic Theory* 4(1): 105–127.

Borzutsky, Silvia. 2006. Cooperation or Confrontation between State and the Market: Social Security and Health Policies. In: Silvia Borzutsky & Lois Hecht Oppenheim (eds.), *After Pinochet: The Chilean Road to Democracy and the Market*. Gainesville: University Press of Florida, pp. 142–166.

Borzutsky, Silvia & Lois Hecht Oppenheim. 2006. Introduction. In: Silvia Borzutsky & Lois Hecht Oppenheim (eds.), *After Pinochet: The Chilean Road to Democracy and the Market*. Gainesville: University Press of Florida, pp. xiiv–xxv.

Canclini, Néstor García. 1989. *Culturas Híbridas: Estrategias para Entrar y Salir de la Modernidad*. Santiago de Chile: Editorial Grijalbo.

Caniuqueo, Sergio. 2006. Siglo XX en Gulumapu: De la fragmentación del Wallmapu a la unidad nacional Mapuche. 1880 a 1978. In: Pablo Marimán, Sergio Caniuqueo, José Millalén, Rodrigo level. Eschucha Winka. Cuatro ensayos de Historia Nacional Mapuche y un epílogo sobre el futuro. Satiago, Lom Ediciones, pp. 129–218.

Caruth, Cathy. 1995. Introduction. In: Cathy Caruth (ed.), *Trauma. Explorations in Memory*. London: Johns Hopkins Press, pp. 3–13.

Caruth, Cathy. 1996. *Unclaimed Experience: Trauma, Narrative, and History*. Baltimore and London: The Johns Hopkins University Press.

Certeau, Michel de. 1984. *The Practice of Everyday Life, trans. by Steven F.* Rendall, Berkeley: University of California.

Chiang, Howard. 2015. Translating culture and psychiatry across the Pacific: How koro became culture bound. *History of Science* 53(1): 102–109.

Citarella, Luca, et al. 1995. *Medicinas y Cultura en la Araucanía*. Santiago de Chile: Editorial Sudamericana.

Coker, Elizabeth Marie. 2004. "Travelling Pains": Embodied Metaphors of Suffering among Southern Sudanese Refugees in Cairo. *Culture, Medicine and Psychiatry* 28: 15–39.

Collier, Simon. 1996. *A History of Chile 1808–1994*. Cambridge: Cambridge University Press.

Collier, Simon & William F. Sater. 2004. *A History of Chile, 1808–2002*. Cambridge: Cambridge University Press.

Comaroff, Jean. 1985. *Body of Power Spirit of Resistance. The Culture and History of a South African People*. Chicago and London: The University of Chicago Press.

Connerton, Paul. 1989. *How Societies Remember*. Cambridge: Cambridge University Press.

Course, Magnus. 2011. *Becoming Mapuche. Person and Ritual in Indigenous Chile*. Chicago: University of Illinois Press.

Crandon-Malamud, Libbet. 1983. Why Susto. *Ethnology. An International Journal of Cultural and Social Anthropology* XXII: 153–169.

Crandon-Malamud, Libbet. 1986. Medical Dialogue and the Political Economy of Medical Pluralism: a Case from Rural Highland Bolivia. *American Ethnologist* 13(3): 463–477.

Crandon-Malamud, Libbet. 1991. *From the Fat of our Souls: Social Change, Political Process, and Medical Pluralism in Bolivia*. Berkeley: University of California Press.

Crandon-Malamud, Libbet. 2003. Changing Times and Changing Symptoms: the Effects of Modernization of Mestizo Medicine in Rural Bolivia (the Case of Two Mestizo Sisters). In: Joan D. Koss-Chioino, Thomas Leatherman & Christine Greenway (eds.), *Medical Pluralism in the Andes*. Psychology Press, pp. 27–42.

Crapanzano, Vincent. 2004. *Imaginative Horizons: An Essay in Literary-philosophical Anthropology*. Chicago and London: University of Chicago Press.

Crow, Joanna. 2013. *The Mapuche in modern Chile: A cultural history*. University Press of Florida.

Cruz-Coke, R. 1992. The Expulsion of the Jesuits (1767) and its impact on Chilean medicine in colonial times. *Rev Med Chil* 120(9): 1062–1069.

Csordas, Thomas. 1988. Embodiment as a Paradigm for Anthropology. *Ethos* 18(1): 5–47. Retrieved from http://www.jstor.org/stable/640395.

Csordas, Thomas. 1994a. *The Sacred Self: A Cultural Phenomenology of Charismatic Healing*. Berkeley and Los Angeles: University of California Press.

Csordas, Thomas. 1994b. Introduction: The Body as Representation and Being-in-the-world. In: Thomas Csordas (ed.), *Embodiment and Experience: The Existential Ground of Culture and Self*. Cambridge: Cambridge University Press, pp. 1–27.

Csordas, Thomas. 1999. The Body's Career in Anthropology. In: Henrietta Moore (ed.), *Anthropological Theory Today*. Cambridge: Polity Press, pp. 193–205.

Csordas, Thomas. 2002 (1988). Embodiment as a Paradigm for Anthropology. In: *Body/Meaning/Healing*. New York: Palgrave Macmillan, pp. 58–88.

Das, Veena & Arthur Kleinman. 2001. Introduction. In: Veena Das, Arthur Kleinman, Margaret Lock, Mamphela Ramphele & Pamela Reynolds (eds.), *Remaking a World: Violence, Social Suffering and Recovery*. Berkeley, Los Angeles, London: University of California Press, pp. 1–31.

De Castro, E.V. 1998. Cosmological deixis and Amerindian perspectivism. *Journal of the Royal Anthropological Institute*: 469–488.

De Castro, E.V. 2004. Exchanging Perspectives: The Transformation of Objects into Subjects in Amerindian Ontologies. *Common Knowledge* 10(3): 463–484.

De Certeau, Michel. 1988. *The Practice of Everyday Life*. Berkeley, Los Angeles, and London: University of California Press.

De la Cadena, M. 2010. Indigenous cosmopolitics in the Andes: Conceptual reflections beyond "politics". *Cultural Anthropology* 25(2): 334–370.

de Moesbach, E.W. & P. Coña. 2000 [1930]. *Vida y costumbres de los indígenas araucanos en la segunda mitad del siglo XIX*. Impr. Cervantes.

Desjarlais, R. 1992. *Body and emotion: The aesthetics of illness and healing in the Nepal Himalayas*. University of Pennsylvania Press.

Desjarlais, R. & C. Jason Throop. 2011. Phenomenological approaches in anthropology. *Annual Review of Anthropology* 40: 87–102.

Desjarlais, Robert, et al. 1995. *World Mental Health: Problems and Priorities in Low-income Countries*. New York: Oxford University Press.

Digiacomo, Susan. 1992. Metaphor as Illness: Postmodern Dilemmas in the Representation of Body, Mind and Disorder. *Medical Anthropology* 14: 109–137.

Dorfman, Ariel. 1985. *A Rural Chilean Legend Come True*. February 18, *New York Times*.

Douglas, Mary. 1970. *Natural Symbols*. Middlesex: Penguin Books.

Dow, J. 1986. Universal Aspects of Symbolic Healing: A Theoretical Synthesis. *American Anthropologist* 88(1): 56–69.

Dowling, Jorge. 1973. *Religión, Chamanismo y Mitología Mapuches*. Santiago de Chile: Editorial Universitaria.

Durkheim, Emile. 1964. *The Elementary Forms of Religious Life*. London: Alden.

Eliade, Mircia. 1964. *Shamanism: Archaic Techniques of Ecstacy*. Bollingen series LXVII. Princeton, NJ: Princeton University Press.

Ellenberger, Henri. 1970. *The Discovery of the Unconscious: The History and Evolution of Dynamic Psychiatry*. New York: Basic Books.

Ercilla, Alonso de. 1982. *Araucania*. Santiago de Chile: Editorial Andres Bello.

Faron, Louis. 1964. *Hawks of the Sun: Mapuche Morality and its Ritual Attributes*. Pittsburgh: University of Pittsburgh Press.

Faron, Louis. 1968. *The Mapuche Indians of Chile*. New York: Holt, Rinehart and Winston.

Faron, Louis. 1969 (1961). *Los Mapuche: Su Estructura Social*. Mexico: Ediciones Especiales.

Fausto, Carlos. 2007. If God were a Jaguar: Cannibalism and Christianity among the Guarai (16th–20th centuries). In: Carlos Fausto & Michael Heckenberger (eds.), *Time and Memory in Indigenous Amazonia; Anthropological Perspectives*. Gainesville: University of Florida Press, pp. 74–105.

Fausto, C. & Heckenberger, M. 2007. *Time and memory in Indigenous Amazonia: anthropological perspectives*. University Press of Florida.

Fernandez, J. 1986. The Argument of Images and the Experience of Returning to the Whole. In: E. Bruner & V. Turner (eds.), *Anthropology of Experience*. Urbana and Chicago: University of Illinois Press, pp. 159–187.

Foerster, Rolf. 1993. *Introducción a la Religiosidad Mapuche*. Santiago de Chile: Editorial Universitaria.

Foerster, Rolf. 1996. *Jesuitas y Mapuches 1593–1767*. Santiago: Editorial Universitaria.

Foerster, Rolf & Sonia Montecino. 1988. *Organizaciones, Líderes y Contiendas Mapuche* (1900–1979). Santiago de Chile: CEM.

Foucault, Michel. 1965 (1988). *Madness and Civilization: A History of Insanity in the Age of Reason*. New York: Vintage Books.

Foucault, Michel. 1977. *Discipline and Punishment. The Birth of the Prison*. New York. Penguin Books.

Foucault, Michel. 1979. *The History of Sexuality. Vol. 1: An Introduction*. London: Penguin Books.

Foucault, Michel. 1980. *Power/Knowledge:* Selected Interviews and other Writings. New York: Pantheon.

Foucault, Michel. 1984. The Politics of Health in the Eighteenth century. In: Paul Rabinow (ed.), *The Foucault Reader*. London: Penguin Books, pp. 273–291.

Foucault, Michel. 1988a. Technologies of the Self. In: M. Luther, Huck Gutman & Patrick Hutton (eds.), *Technolgies of the Self: A Seminar with Michel Foucault*. Amherst: The University of Massachusetts Press, pp. 16–50.

Foucault, Michel. 1988b. *The History of Sexuality. Vol. 3. The Care of the Self.* London: Allen Lane.

Foucault, Michel. 1994 (1973). *The Birth of the Clinic: An Archaeology of Medical Perception*. New York: Vintage Books.

Freud, Sigmund. 1919 (1955). The 'Uncanny' [*Das unheimliche*]. From Standard Edition, Vol. XVII, trans. James Strachey. London: Hogarth Press, pp. 217–256.

Geschiere, Peter. 1997. *The Modernity of Witchcraft: Politics and the Occult in Postcolonial Africa*. Charlottesville: The University of Virginia Press.

Giaconi, Juan. 1994. Proyecciones de las reformas introducidos en el sector de salud durante el Gobierno de las Fuerzas Armadas (1973–1990). In: Ernesto Miranda (ed.), *La Salud en Chile. Evolucion y Perspectivas*. Santiago de Chile: Centro de Estudios Publicos, pp. 257–273.

Gillen, J. 1948. Magical Fright. *Psychiatry* 11(4): 387–400.

Giminiani, Piergiorgio Di. 2012. *Tierras ancestrales, disputas contemporáneas. Perteninencia y demandas territoriales en la sociedad mapuche rural.* Santiago: Ediciones Universidad Católica de Chile.

Gluckman, M. 1958. *Analysis of a Social Situation in Modern Zululand*. The Rhodes-Livingstone papers, number twenty-eight. New York: Manchester University Press.

Gluckman, M. 2006. Ethnographic Data in British Social Anthropology. In: T.M.S. Evens & Don Handelman (eds.), *The Manchester School: Practice and Ethnographic Praxis in Anthropology*. New York and Oxford: Berghahn Books, pp. 13–25.

Gobierno de Chile, Ministerio de Salud. 2003. *Resultados I Encuesta de salud, Chile 2003*. Gobierno de Chile, Ministerio de Salud.

Gonzales Galves, Marcelo Ignacio. 2012. Personal Truths, Shared Equivocations. Otherness, Uniqueness, and Social Life among the Mapuche of Southern Chile. PhD in Social Anthropology. The University of Edinburgh.

Gonzales Galves, Marcelo Ignacio. 2015. The truth of experience and its communication: Reflections on Mapuche epistemology. *Anthropological Theory* 15(2): 141–157.

Good, Byron J. 1996. Culture and DSM-IV: Diagnosis, Knowledge and Power. *Culture, Medicine and Psychiatry* 20: 127–132.

Good, Byron J. 1997. Studying Mental Illness in Context: Local, Global, or Universal? *Ethos* 25(2): 230–248.

Grebe, María Ester. 1972. La Cosmovisión Mapuche. *Cuadernos de la Realidad Nacional* 14: 46–74.

Guarnaccia, Peter. 1993. Ataques de Nervios in Puerto Rico: Culture-Bound Syndromes or Popular Illness. *Medical Anthropology* 15: 157–1965.

Guarnaccia, Peter. 2003. Editorial. *Culture, Medicine and Psychiatry* 27: 249–257.

Guevara, Tomas. 1913. Las Ultimas Familas y Costumbres Araucanas. Santiago: Imprente, Litografía I Encuadernacion "Barcelona".

Hacking, Ian. 1995. *Rewriting the Soul: Multiple Personality and the Sciences of Memory*. Princeton, NJ: Princeton University Press.

Hacking, Ian. 1996. Memory Sciences, Memory Politics. In: Paul Antze & Michael Lambek (eds.), *Tense Past: Cultural Essays in Trauma and Memory*. New York: Routledge, pp. 67–89.

Halbwachs, Maurice. 1992. *On Collective Memory*. London: University of Chicago Press.

Han, Clara. 2004. The Work of Indebtedness: The Traumatic Present of Late Capitalist Chile. *Culture, Medicine and Psychiatry* 28(2): 169–187.

Han, Clara. 2012. *Life in Debt. Times of Care and Violence in Neoliberal Chile*. London: University of California Press.

Henare, Amiria, Martin Holbraad & Sari Wastell. 2007. Introduction. In: A. Henare, M. Holbraad & S. Wastell (eds.), *Thinking through Things: Theorising Artefact Ethnographically*. London: Routledge, pp. 1–32.

ILAS, Instituto Latinamericano de Salud Mental y Derechos Humanos. 1996. *Reparación Derechos Humanos y Salud Mental*. Santiago de Chile: ediciones Chile America CESOC.

Inostroza, I. 2011. La agricultura en las comunidades Mapuches de Chile 1850–1890.

Instituto de Estudios Indigenas. 2003. *Los Derechos de los Pueblos Indígenas en Chile: Informe de Programa de Derechos Indígenas.* Universidad de la Frontera Temuco: Lom Ediciones.

Jackson, Michael. 2002. *The Politics of Storytelling: Violence, Transgression, and Intersubjectivity.* Copenhagen: Museum Tusculanum Press.

Janzen, John. 1978. *The Quest for Therapy: Medical Pluralism in Lower Zaire.* Berkeley, Los Angeles, and London: University of California Press.

Janzen, John. 2002. *The Social Fabric of Health: An Introduction to Medical Anthropology.* New York: McGraw-Hill.

Johannessen, Helle. 2005. Body and Self in Medical Pluralism. In: Helle Johanessen & Imre Lázár (eds.), *Multiple Medical Realities: Patients and Healers in Biomedical, Alternative and Traditional Medicine.* Oxford and New York: Berghahn, pp. 1–21.

Johansen, Katrine Schepelern. 2006. *Kultur og Psykiatri: En Antropologi om Transkulturel Psykiatri på Danske Hospitaler.* Ph.D.- afhandling. København: Institut for Antropologi og Sct. Hans Hospital.

Johnson, Mark. *The Body in the Mind: The Bodily Basis of Meaning, Imagination, and Reason.*

Jones, Kristine. 1999. The Southern Margin (1673–1882). In: Frank Salomon & Stuart Schwartz (eds.), *The Cambridge History of Native People of the Americas.* Volume 3, South America part 2. New York. Cambridge University Press, pp. 140–181.

Kaiser, B.N., E.E. Haroz, B.A. Kohrt, P.A. Bolton, J.K. Bass & D.E. Hinton 2015. "Thinking too much": A systematic review of a common idiom of distress. *Social Science & Medicine* 147: 170–183.

Kapferer, Bruce. 1987. The Anthropology of Max Gluckman. *Social Analysis* 22: 3–21.

Kapferer, Bruce. 1997. *The Feast of the Sorcerer. Practices of Consciousness and Power.* Chicago: Chicago University Press.

Kapferer, Bruce. 2003. Sorcery, Modernity and the Constitutive Imaginary: Hybridising Continuities. In: Bruce Kapferer (ed.), *Beyond Rationalism: Rethinking Magic, Witchcraft and Sorcery.* London and New York: Berghahn Books, pp. 105–128.

Kapferer, Bruce. 2006. Situations, Crisis, and the Anthropology of the Concrete: The Contribution of Max Gluckman. In: T.M.S. & Don Handelman (eds.), *The Manchester School: Practice and Ethnographic Praxis in Anthropology.* Oxford and New York, pp. 118–159.

Kelly, José Antonio. 2011. *State Healthcare and Yanomamo Transformation. A symmetrical Ethnography.* Tucson: University of Arizona Press.

Kempny, Marian. 2006. History of the Manchester "School" and the Extended-Case Method. *Social Analysis* 49(3): 144–165.

Kirmayer, Lawrence. 1988. Mind and Body as Hidden Values in Biomedicine. In: M. Lock & D.R. Gorden (eds.), *Biomedicine Examined*. Dordrecht: Kluwer Academic Publishers, pp. 57–93.

Kirmayer, Lawrence. 1992. The Body's Insistence of Meaning: Metaphor as Presentations and Representations in Illness Experience. *Medical Anthropology Quarterly, New Series* 6(4): 323–346.

Kirmayer, Lawrence. 1996. Landscapes of Memory: Trauma, Narrative, and Dissociation. In: Paul Antze & Michael Lambek (eds.), *Tense Past: Cultural Essays in Trauma and Memory*. New York: Routledge, pp. 173–199.

Kirmayer, Lawrence. 2000. Broken Narratives: Clinical Encounters and the Poetics of Illness Experience. In: Cheryl Mattingly & Linda Carro (eds.), *Narrative and the Cultural Construction of Illness and Healing*. London: University of California Press, pp. 153–181.

Kirmayer, Lawrence. 2004. Explaining Medically Unexplained Symptoms. *Canadian Journal of Psychiatry* 49(10): 663–672.

Kirmayer, Lawrence & Allan Young. 1998. Culture and Somatization: Clinical, Epidemiological, and Ethnographic Perspective. *Psychosomatic Medicine* 60(4): 420–431.

Kirmayer, L. J., & Young, A. 1998. Culture and somatization: clinical, epidemiological, and ethnographic perspectives. *Psychosomatic medicine* 60(4): 420–430.

Kirmayer, Lawrence & Noman Sartorius. 2007. Cultural Models and Somatic Syndromes. *Psychosomatic Medicines* 69: 832–840.

Kleinman, Arthur. 1978. Concepts and a Model for the Comparison of Medical Systems as Cultural Systems. *Social Science and Medicine* 1: 85–93.

Kleinman, Arthur. 1980. *Patients and Healers in the Context of Culture: An Exploration of the Borderland between Anthropology, Medicine and Psychiatry*. Berkeley: University of California Press.

Kleinman, Arthur. 1986. *Social Origins of Distress and Disease: Depression, Neurasthenia, and Pain in Modern China*. New Haven: Yale University Press.

Kleinman, Arthur. 1994. How Bodies Remember: Social Memory and Bodily Experience of Criticism, Resistance and Delegitimation following China's Cultural Revolution. *New Literary History* 25(3), 25th Anniversary Issue: 707–723.

Kleinman, Arthur & Anne E. Becker. 1998. "Sociosomatics": The Contributions of Anthropology to Psychosomatic Medicine. *Journal of the American Psychosomatic Society* 60(4): 389–394.

Kohrt, Brandon A., Emily Mendenhall & Peter J. Brown. 2016. Historical Background: Medical Anthropology and Global Mental Health. *Global Mental Health: Anthropological Perspectives*. Routledge.

Kohrt, B.A., D.J. Hruschka, H.E. Kohrt, N.L. Panebianco & G. Tsagaankhuu 2004. Distribution of distress in post-socialist Mongolia: a cultural epidemiology of yadargaa. *Social Science & Medicine* 58(3): 471–485.

Koss, Chionino, Leatherman T. & Christine Greenway (eds.). 2003. *Medical Pluralism in the Andes*. Psychology Press.

Kristensen, Dorthe Brogård. 1999. Chile. In: *The Indigenous World 1998–1999*. København: Iwgia, pp. 121–124.

Kristensen, Dorthe Brogård. 2000. Chile. In: *The Indigenous World 1999–2000*. København: Iwgia, pp. 142–148.

Kristensen, Dorthe Brogård. 2001. Chile. In: *The Indigenous World 2000–2001*. København: Iwgia, pp. 161–167.

Kristensen Benedikte, Møller. 2015. *Returning to the Forest: Shamanism, Landscape and History among the Duha of Northern Mongolia*. PhD thesis University of Copenhagen.

Kuramocho, Yosuke. 1991. *Mitología Mauche. Colección 500 años*. Quito: Abya-Yala.

Lambek, Michael. 1996. The Past Imperfect: Remembering as Moral Practice. In: Paul Antze & Michael Lambek (eds.), *Tense Past: Cultural Essays in Trauma and Memory*. New York: Routledge, pp. 235–254.

Latcham, Ricardo. 1924. *La Organización Social y las Creencias Religiopsas de los Antiguos Araucanos*. Santiago de Chile: Imprenta Cervante.

Latcham, Ricardo. 1928. *La Prehistoria Chilena*. Santiago de Chile: Soc. Imp. Y Lit. Universo.

Leder, Drew. 1990. *The Absent Body*. Chicago and London: Chicago University Press.

Lévi-Strauss, Claude. 1968. *The Origin of the Table Manners: Introduction to a Science of Mythology*. New York: Basic Books.

Lévi-Strauss, Claude. 2000 (1949). The Effectiveness of Symbols. In: Roland Littlewood & Simon Dein (eds.), *Cultural Psychiatry and Medical Anthropology: An Introduction and Reader*. London and New Brunswick: The Athlone Press, pp. 162–177.

Lewis-Fernandéz, R. 1996. Cultural Formulation of Psychiatric Diagnosis: Introduction. *Culture, Medicine and Psychiatry* 20: 133–144.

Lincoqueo, José Huenuman. 2002. Genocidio, Cabello de Troya de Mefistífeles (El Demonios). Análisis Jurídico acerca de los Parlamentos. In: Carlos Contreras Painemal (ed.), *Actas del Primer Congreso Internacional de Historia Mapuche*. UKE Mapuförlaget, pp. 70–76.

Lindhardt, M. 2012. Power in powerlessness: a study of Pentecostal life worlds in urban Chile (Vol. 12). Brill.

Lindhardt, Martin. 2004. *Power in Powerlessness: A Study of Pentacostal Life Worlds Urban Chile*. PhD Thesis. Institut for Etnografi og social antropologi, Århus Universitet.

Littlewood, Roland & Simon Dein (eds.). 2000. Introduction. In: Roland Littlewood & Simon Dein (eds.), *Cultural Psychiatry and Medical Anthropology: An Introduction and Reader*. London and New Brunswick: The Athlone Press, pp. 1–34.

Lock, Margaret. 1993. Cultivating the Body: Anthropological and Epistemologies of Bodily Practices and Knowledge. *Annual Review of Anthropology*. 1993: 133–155.

Lock, Margaret & Nancy Scheper-Hughes. 1990. A Critical-Interpretive Approach in Medical Anthropology: Rituals and Routines of Discipline and Dissent. In: Thomas M. Johnson and Carolyn Fishel Sargent (eds.), *Medical Anthropology, Contemporary Theory and Method*. Westport: Praeger Publishers, pp. 47–73.

Lock, Margaret & Nancy Scheper-Hughes. 1996. A Critical-Interpretive Approach in Medical Anthropology: Rituals and Routines of Discipline and Dissent. In: Carolyn Fishel Sargent and Thomas M. Johnson (eds.), *Medical Anthropology, Contemporary Theory and Method*. Westport: Praeger Publishers, Rev. ed., pp. 41–70.

Loveman, Brian. 2001. *Chile: The Legacy of Hispanic Capitalism*. New York and Oxford: Oxford University Press.

Low, Setha. 1988. Medical Practice in Response to a Folk Illness: The Diagnosis and Treatment of *Nervios* in Costa Rica. In: M. Lock & D.R. Gordon (eds.), *Biomedicine Examined*. Dordrecht: Kluwer Academic Publishers, 415–438.

Low, Setha. 1994. Embodied Metaphors: Nerves as Lived Experience. In: Thomas Csordas (ed.), *Embodiment and Experience*. Cambridge: Cambridge University Press, pp. 139–162.

Luna, L. 2007. *Un mundo entre dos mundos: las relaciones entre el pueblo mapuche y el estado chileno desde la perspectiva del desarrollo y de los cambios socioculturales*. Sede Villarrica: Pontificia Universidad Católica de Chile.

Mai, F. 2004. Somatization disorder: a practical review. *The Canadian Journal of Psychiatry* 49(10): 652–662.

Mallon, F.E. 2005. *Courage tastes of blood: The Mapuche community of Nicolás Ailío and the Chilean state, 1906–2001*. Duke University Press.

Marcus, George. 1995. Ethnography in/Of the World System: The Emergence of Multi-Sited Ethnography. *Annual Reviews* 24: 95–117.

Marimán, Pablo. 2006. Los mapuche antes de la conquista militar chileno-argentina. In: Pablo Marimán, Sergio Caniuqueo, José Millalén, Rodrigo level. Eschucha Winka. Cuatro ensayos de Historia Nacional Mapuche y un epílogo sobre el futuro. Satiago: Lom Ediciones, pp. 53–128.

Mariqueo, Reynaldo. 1989. *The Etno-Development of the Mapuche People*. IWGIA document no. 63. IWGIA: Copenhagen.

Merleau-Ponty, Maurice. 1962. *Phenomenology of Perception*. London and New York: Routledge.

Merleau-Ponty, Maurice. 2002. *Phenomenology of Perception*. London and New York: Routledge.

Miles, Ann & Thomas Leatherman. 2003. Perspectives on Medical Anthropology in the Andes. In: Joan D. Koss-Chioino, Thomas Leatherman & Christine Greenway (eds.), *Medical Pluralism in the Andes*. Psychology Press, pp. 3–16.

Ministerio del Interior de Chile. 2003. Decreto n.° 19: Comisión Verdad y Nuevo Trato, *Biblioteca del Congreso Nacional de Chile*.

Ministerio de Salud, Gobierno de Chile. 1998. *Diagnostico y tratamiento de la depresion en nivel primario de Atencion. Dept. programas de las personas*. Unidad de Salud Mental. Serie MINSAL 03- Guias Metodológicas SM no.3.

Ministerio de Salud [Minsal]. 2006. *Avances de la salud en Chile*.

Ministerio de Salud & Gobierno de Chile. 2000. Guá Clínica para la Atención Primaria. La depression, Detección, Diagnóstico y Tratamiento. DISAP Unidad de Salud mental.

Minsal. Gobierno de Chile, Ministerio de Salud. 2003. *Resultados 1 Encuesta de Salud*.

Minsal. Gobierno de Chile, Ministerio de Salud. 2017. *Encuesta Nacional de Salud 2016–2017*. Primeros resultados.

Miranda, Ernesto (ed.). 1994. *La salud en Chile: Evolucion y perspectivas*. Santiago de Chile: Centro de Estudios Publicos.

Montecino, Sonia. 1985. *Mujeres Mapuche: El Saber Tradicional de la Curación de Enfermedades Communes*. Santiago de Chile: CEM.

Montecino, Sonia. 1996. *Madres y Huachos: Alegorías del Mestizaje Chileno*. Santiago: Biblioteca Claves de Chile. Editorial Sudamericana.

Montecino, Sonia. 1999. *Sueño con Menguante: Biografía de una Machi*. Santiago de Chile: Editorial Sudamericana.

Montecino, Sonia. 2003. *Mitos de Chile: Diccionario de Seres, Magia y Encantos*. Santiago de Chile: Editorial Sudamericana.

Moulian, Tomás. 1997. *Anatomía de un Mito*. Arcis Universidad: LOM Ediciones, Serie Punto de Fga. Coleccion sin Norte.

Mysik, Avis. 1998. Susto: An Illness of the Poor. *Dialectical Anthropology* 23: 187–202.

Nájera, Alfonso Gonzáles de. 1971. *Desengaño y reparo de la guerra del reino de Chile*. Santiago de Chile: Editorial Andres Bello.

Nichter, Mark. 1981. Idioms of Distress: Alternatives in the Expression of Psychosocial Distress: A Case Study from South India. *Culture, Medicine and Psychiatry* 5: 379–408.

Nichter, Mark & Margaret Lock (eds.). 2002. Introduction: from Documenting Medical Pluralism to Critical Interpretations of Globalized Health Knowledge, Policies and Practices. In: Mark Nichter & Margaret Lock (eds.), *New Horizons in Medical Anthropology*, pp. 1–35.

Núñez de Pineda, F. 1863. *Cautiverio feliz y razón de las guerras dilatadas de Chile*. Santiago: Imprenta de Ferrocarril (Obra original publicada en 1673).

Organización Panamericana de la Salud. 2002. *La salud pública y la organizacion panamericana de la salud en Chile (1902–2002). Cien años de colaboración.* Santiago de Chile: Organización panamericana de la Salud.

Ovalle, Alonso de. 2003 (1646). *Historia relacion del reino de Chile.* Santiago de Chile: Pehuén. Biblioteca del Bicentenario.

Painemal, Carlos Contreras. 2002. Actas del Primer Congreso Internacional de Historia Mapuche. ÑUKE Mapuförlaget.

Pairican, Fernando Padilla. 2012. Sembrando ideología: el Aukiñ Wallmapu Ngulam in the transition of Aylwin (1990–1994). *Sudhistoria* 4: 12–42.

Pairican, Fernando Padilla. 2015. El retorno de un viejo actor político: el guerrero. Perspectivas para comprender la violencia política en el movimiento mapuche (1990–2010). In *Violencia coloniales en Wallmapu.* Centro de Estudios y Investigaciones Mapuche, pp. 301–324.

Paley, Julia. 2001. *Marketing Democracy: Power and Social Movements in Post-dictatorship Chile.* London: University of California Press.

Panter-Brick, C. & Eggerman, M. 2017. *Anthropology and Global Mental Health: Depth, Breadth, and Relevance.* In: White R., Jain S., Orr D. & Read U. (eds.), *The Palgrave Handbook of Sociocultural Perspectives on Global Mental Health.* London: Palgrave Macmillan.

Parker, Cristián. 1996. *Popular Religion & Modernization in Latin America. A Different Logic.* New York: Orbis Books.

Patel, V. 2012. Global mental health: from science to action. *Harvard Review of Psychiatry* 20(1): 6–12.

Pérez, Gabriela. 2000. Población Mapuche en Chile. Situación sociodemográfica. Censo de 1992. In: Sandrá Pérez Infante (ed.), *Pueblo Mapuche: desarollo y autogestón. Análisis y perspectives en une sociedad pluricultural.* Conception: escaparate Ediciones, pp. 61–79.

Petersen, Morten Axel. 2011. *Not quite Shamans. Spirit Worlds and Political Lives in Northern Mongolia.* New York: Cornell Press.

Pineda y Bascuñan, Franscisco. 1863. *El cautiverio feliz y razon de las guerras dilatadas de Chile.* Santiago de Chile: Imprenta del Ferrocaril.

Pinto, Jorge. 1988. *Misioneros en la Araucania 1600–1900.* Temuco: Ediciones Universaidad de la frontera, Serie quinto centenario.

Pinto, Jorge. 2000. *De la inclusión a la exclusión. La formación del estado, la nación y el pueblo mapuche.* Santiago: Universidad de Santiago.

Pizza, Giovianni. 2005. *Saperi, partiche e politiche del corpo.* Roma: Carocci.

Pizza, Giovianni. 2006. *Antonio Gramsci and Medical Anthropology Now: Hegemony, Agency, and Transforming Persons.* English translation of the article: "Antonio Gramsci e l'antropologia medica ora. Egemonia, agentività e trasformazioni della persona. AM. Rivista della Società italiana di antropologia medica", n 15–16, ottobre 2003.

PNUD. 2000. *Desarrollo humano en Chile 2000: Mas sociedad para gobernar el futuro.*

Quaranta, Ivo. 2001. Contextualising the Body: Anthropology, Biomedicine and Medical Anthropology. *Rivista Della Societá Italiana Di Antropología Medica* 11–12: 155–171.

Rahier, Jean Muteba. 2003. Introduction: *Mestizaje, Mulataje, Mestiçagem* in Latin American Ideologies of National Identities. *Journal of Latin American Anthropology* 8(1): 40–51.

Richards, P. 2010. Of Indians and terrorists: how the state and local elites construct the Mapuche in neoliberal multicultural Chile. *Journal of Latin American Studies* 42(1): 59–90.

Richards, P. 2013. *Race and the Chilean miracle: Neoliberalism, democracy, and indigenous rights.* University of Pittsburgh Press.

Ronald C. Simons & Charles C. Hughes. 1986. *The culture-bound syndromes: Folk illnesses of psychiatric and anthropological interest.* In: Ronald C. Simons & Charles C. Hughes (eds.). The Netherlands: D. Reidel.

Rønsbo, Henrik. 2008. Hybridity and Change: Gamonales, Monteneros and Young Politicos in SouthCentral Peru. *Bullitin of Latin American Research* 27:83.

Rosales, Diego. 1989 (1674). *Historia general del reino de Chile.* Valparaiso: Imprenta de El Mercurio.

Rose, Nicolas. 1999. *Governing the Soul: The Shaping of the Private Self.* London and New York: Free Association Books.

Rose, Nicolas. 2006. Governing "Advanced" Liberal Democracies. In: Aradhana Sharma & Akhil Gupta (eds.), *The Anthropology of the State.* Malden and Oxford: Blackwell Publishing.

Rubel, A. 1964. The Epidemiology of a Folk Illness: Susto in Hispanic America. *Ethnology* 3: 268–283.

Rubel, Arthur, O'Nell Carl & Rolando Collado-Ardón. 1984. *Susto: A Folk Illness.* Berkeley and Los Angeles: University of California Press.

Salazar, Gabriel & Julio Pinto. 1999. *Historia contemporánea de Chile II: Actores, identidad y movimiento.* Santiago: LOM Ediciones.

Saldivia, Sandra, et al. 2004. Use of Mental Health Services in Chile. *Psychiatric Services* 55: 71–76.

Schamis, Hector E. 1999. *Reforming the State: The Politics of Privatization in Latin America and Europe.* Ann Arbor: The University of Michigan Press.

Scheper-Hughes, N. 1993. *Death without weeping: The violence of everyday life in Brazil.* Berkeley: University of California Press.

Scheper-Hughes, N. 1994. Embodied Knowledge: Thinking with the Body in Critical Medical Anthropology. In: Robert Borofsky (ed.), *Assessing Cultural Anthropology.* New York: McGraw-Hill, pp. 229–241.

Scheper-Hughes, Nancy & Margaret Lock. 1987. The Mindful Body: A Prolegomenon to Future Work in Medical Anthropology. *Medical Anthropology Quarterly* 1(1): 6–41.

Simons, Ronald & Charles Hughes (eds.). 1985. *The Culture-Bound Syndromes: Folk Illnesses of Psychiatric and Anthropological Interest.* Dordrecth: D. Reidel Publishing Company.

Sontag, Susan. 1991. *Illness as Metaphor: Aids and its Metaphors.* London: Penguin Books.

Stavenhagen, Rodolfo. 2003. Informe del Relator Especial sobre la situación de los derechos humanos y las libertades fundamentales de los indígenas, presentado de conformidad con la resolución 2003/56 de la Comisión.

Stern, Steve. 2006a. *Remembering Pinochet's Chile: On the Eve of London 1998.* Book One of the Trilogy: The Memory Box of Pinochet's Chile. Durham: Duke University Press.

Stern, Steve. 2006b. *Battling for Hearts and Minds: Memory Struggle in Pinochet's Chile, 1973–1988.* Book Two of the Trilogy: The Memory Box of Pinochet's Chile. Durham: Duke University Press.

Stewart, Carmen López. 2004. Chile Mental Health Country Profile. *International Review of Psychiatry* 16(1–2): 73–82.

Stoller, Paul. 1984. Horrific comedy: cultural resistance and Songhay possession dance. *Ethos* 11:165–187.

Stoller, Paul. 1989. *Fusion of the Worlds: an Ethnography of Possession Among the Songhay of Niger.* Chicago: University of Chicago Press.

Stoller, Paul. 1995. *Embodying Colonial Memories: Spirit Possession, Power, and the Hauka in West Africa.* New York and London: Routledge.

Taussig, Michael. 1980. *The Devil and Commodity Fetishism in South America.* Chapel Hill: The University of North Carolina Press.

Taussig, Michael. 1987. *Shamanism, Colonialism and the Wild Man.* Chicago and London: The University of Chicago Press.

Taussig, Michael. 1992. Reification and the Consciousness of the Patient. In: Michael Taussig (ed.), *The Nervous System.* New York and London: Routledge, pp. 83–111.

Taussig, Michael. 1993. *Mimesis and Alterity. A Particular History of the Senses.* New York: Routledge.

Taussig, Michael. 1999. *Defacement. Public Secrecy and the Labor of the Negative.* Stanford: Sanford University Press.

Taylor, Anne-Christine. 2007. Sick of History: Contrasting regimes of Historicity in the Upper Amazonian. In: Carlos Fausto & Michael Heckenberger (eds.), *Time and Memory in Indigenous Amazonia; Anthropological Perspectives.* Gainesville: University of Florida Press, pp. 133–168.

Torri, Maria Costanza. 2012. Intercultural Health Practices: Towards an Equal Recognition Between Indigenous Medicine and Biomedicine? A case study from Chile. *Health care Anal* 20: 31–49.

Turner, Brian. 1992. *Regulating Bodies: Essays in Medical Sociology.* London and New York: Routledge.

Turner, Brian. 1996. *The Body and Society: Explorations in Social Theory*. London: Sage Publications.

Turner, Victor. 1957. *Schism and Continuity in an African Society: A Study of Ndembu Village Life*. Manchester: Manchester University Press.

Turner, Victor. 1967. *Forest of Symbols: Aspects of Ndembu Ritual*. Ithaca, NY: Cornell University Press.

Turner, Victor. 1974. *Dramas, Fields and Metaphors*. Ithaca, NY: Cornell University Press.

Valdivia, Luis. 1621. Sermon en lengva de Chile, de los mysterios de nvestra santa fe catholica, para dedicarla a los indios infieles del reyno de Chile, dividido en nveve partes pequeñas, acomodadas a fu capacidad.

van der Kolk, Bessel A. & Onno van der Hart. 1995. The intrusive Past: The Flexibility of Memory and the Engraving of Trauma. In: Cathy Caruth (ed.), *Trauma, Explorations in Memory*. Baltimore and London: The Johns Hopkins University Press, pp. 158–183.

Van Velsen, J. 1967. The Extended-case Method and Situational Analysis. In: A.L. Epstein (ed.), *The Craft of Social Anthropology*. London: Tavistock, pp. 129–149.

Villalobos, Sergio. 1995. Vida Fronteriza de la Ataucania. El Mito de la Guerra de Arauco. Santiago: Editional Andres Bello.

WHO. 2001. *The World Health Report 2001. Mental Health: New Understanding, New Hope*. Geneva: WHO.

Yap, P.M. 2001 (1951). Mental Diseases Peculiar to Certain Culture: a Survey of Comparative Psychiatry. In: Roland Littlewood & Simon Dein (eds.), *Cultural Psychiatry and Medical Anthropology: An Introduction and Reader*. London and New Brunswick: The Athlone Press, pp. 179–198.

Yarris, K. 2016. Grandmothers, Children, and Intergenerational Distress in Nicaraguan Transnational Families. In: Brandon A. Kohrt, Emily Mendenhall & Peter J. Brown (eds.), *Global Mental Health*. Routledge, pp. 117–134.

Young, Allan. 1995. *The Harmony of Illusions: Inventing Post-Traumatic Stress Disorder*. Princeton, NJ: Princeton University Press.

Young, Allan. 1996. Bodily Memory and Traumatic memory. In: Paul Antze & Michael Lambek (eds.), *Tense Past: Cultural Essays in Trauma and Memory*. New York: Routledge, pp. 89–103.

AUTHOR INDEX[1]

[1] Note: Page numbers followed by 'n' refer to notes.

© The Author(s) 2019
D. B. Kristensen, *Patients, Doctors and Healers*,
https://doi.org/10.1007/978-3-319-97031-8

Subject Index[1]

[1] Note: Page numbers followed by 'n' refer to notes.

© The Author(s) 2019   225
D. B. Kristensen, *Patients, Doctors and Healers*,
https://doi.org/10.1007/978-3-319-97031-8

The manufacturer's authorised representative in the EU is Springer
Nature Customer Service Centre GmbH, Europaplatz 3, 69115 Heidelberg,
Germany. If you have any concerns regarding our products, please
contact ProductSafety@springernature.com

Printed and bound by CPI Group (UK) Ltd, Croydon, CR0 4YY
27/04/2026
02097570-0001